PROVIDER-LED
POPULATION
HEALTH MANAGEMENT

KEY STRATEGIES FOR HEALTHCARE
IN THE NEXT TRANSFORMATION

RICHARD HODACH, MD, MPH, PhD

authorHOUSE®

AuthorHouse™
1663 Liberty Drive
Bloomington, IN 47403
www.authorhouse.com
Phone: 1-800-839-8640

Published by AuthorHouse   01/06/2015

ISBN: 978-1-4969-4174-9 (sc)
ISBN: 978-1-4969-4175-6 (hc)
ISBN: 978-1-4969-4173-2 (e)

Library of Congress Control Number: 2014917357

This book is printed on acid-free paper.

Contents

Section 3   Implementing Change

Foreword

As the founding Dean of the nation's only school of Population Health, I am always interested in new books in our field. This is especially true because, regrettably, there is confusion in the marketplace about the term "population health" and the future of our field. Fortunately, along comes Dr. Richard Hodach and his colleagues at Phytel in their new book, "Provider-Led Population Health Management." Even the title had me very intrigued.

"Provider-Led Population Health Management" means just that! To me it is an explicit recognition of the powerful cultural change we must implement in order for clinicians to lead a population health revolution. Hodach has given us just the tools we need to lead such a revolution.

This book connects the dots. It takes the components of population health management, such as Accountable Care Organizations, patient-centered medical homes, pay-for-performance contracts, and clearly articulates expert definitions. It is the best description of these tools that I have seen. The book raises an important question, namely, how can we distill the lessons from leading population health organizations such as Kaiser Permanente, Geisinger, and others and diffuse these lessons more broadly into the healthcare system? I believe Dr. Hodach has outlined exactly how we might tackle this challenge.

For example, in the chapter dealing with clinically integrated networks, Hodach recognizes that to be effective, these networks must deploy and connect care managers, engage with all patients, especially those recently discharged from the hospital and measure provider performance. Only a book focused on provider-led population health management could connect all these dots with a special emphasis on clinician self-reflection and provider outcome measurement. Sure, the information technology is the circulatory system to make these programs really work effectively, but Hodach recognizes that it's much more than getting the "wires" right, it's getting the cultural change that we really need!

Another particular strength of the book is the wonderful description of meaningful use, both current manifestations and predicted in the near term. For example, Stage 3 meaningful use in the proposed mandates, must promote patient engagement and patients must be able to download their own laboratory tests within 24 hours. This is a sea change in how providers and patients will interact in the very near future. I am moved to ask, what has the nation gained by the $23 billon the government has spent in incentives toward implementing meaningful use? Maybe the answer lies in Stage 3 mandates.

Two other sections of the book really blew me away! The section on the return on investment of change and the implementation of lean thinking as a core component of the patient engagement strategy are first rate. "Lean" is not just a course or a CME event, "lean" is the critical strategy driving patient engagement and we know without patient engagement, we simply can't improve the health of the population. Hodach lays it all out and once again connects those dots.

As far as those patient-centered medical homes and all the recent controversy regarding the evidence about their effectiveness, Hodach gets right to the point. To perform population health management effectively, the patient-centered medical home must use information technology to coordinate care, create registries and once again, engage with patients. I could not have said it better myself.

Kudos to Hodach and the entire team at Phytel. No one, including me, presumes that one information technology firm can change the world, but clearly our colleagues at Phytel have laid the groundwork for a new view of population health—one that is led by providers.

I'm confident that this book will be widely read and more importantly, used every day to improve the health of our population. As a Dean, I'm anxious to make this book part of our scholarly armamentarium!

Hodach has shown us how to clearly connect the dots and change the culture. The question remains, are we able to embrace his message?

David B. Nash, MD, MBA
Founding Dean
Jefferson School of Population Health

Preface: A Journey to Health

In 2008, I was named Chief Executive Officer of Phytel with the charge to lead the company in a new direction. I saw the emerging and rising interest in quality metrics, value-based payment and population health management. I proceeded to write a business plan laying out the opportunity for the company and the steps we would take to prepare Phytel to seize the day. Or as Wayne Gretzky says, "I skate to where the puck is going to be, not where it has been." And that thought characterized how the Phytel team approached the work of innovating and building the next generation of products in preparation for the anticipated shift in the healthcare market.

Having previously founded and led one of the country's very first disease management companies, I knew the transition ahead would require a combination of creative thinking, forethought, and persistent leadership to overcome certain common challenges. Chief among these, in my mind, is how to encourage patients affected by chronic conditions or in need of recommended care to consistently engage with their physicians to attend to their healthcare needs. It's clear that when patients who have stopped seeing their doctor re-engage with their provider, a lot of good things can happen. Ultimately, better and more proactive management of health requires individuals to change health behaviors. But to get there, the person must engage and have the right dialogue and relationship with their doctor and care team.

One key to driving behavior change is tailored education that addresses a person's knowledge deficits about their condition. Professional educators know that people have a tendency to learn in different ways. Some are visual learners, some are auditory, and some only learn by *doing*. Clayton Christensen, the thought-leader behind disruptive innovation, pushed this idea into the information age with his book, *The Disruptive Classroom*. Christensen proposed using technology to match a given curriculum with the unique teaching styles needed to reach the different types of learners.

Today at Phytel, we are incorporating many of these learning insights but applied and fine-tuned for the world of healthcare. We provide our physician clients with a variety of multi-modal communication tools and workflow-friendly technologies designed to identify patients with critical care gaps, reach out to them in the manner that's most effective (phone, email, text, etc.), engage them, and then track their responses so we know what works and what doesn't work for different cohorts. Then we refine and repeat the process. In this way, we are helping physician organizations across the country build stronger relationships with their most at-risk patients, and helping patients maintain and improve their overall health. It's the full-spectrum solution to population health management that I have personally been striving to realize for many years.

In this preface, I want to tell you a little about my quest, and then explain why I think the book you're holding in your hands right now is the key to understanding how your healthcare organization can succeed in the new world of healthcare.

***

Following an insightful and rewarding few years teaching and coaching after college, I was recruited into medical sales by a company that would later become part of Baxter. I eventually joined a startup consulting company called Quantum Health Resources that would later conduct an IPO and become a very successful public company.

Quantum, which focused on providing drugs and services for hemophiliacs, was the perfect place for my interests. In my years there I saw true entrepreneurism constantly on display and learned the fundamentals of building a successful business from my boss and mentor, the late Doug Stickney, Quantum's impassioned entrepreneur-CEO. One of Doug's CEO dictums that I still follow today is, "You don't have to know all the answers yourself, but you do need to lead processes to get all of the answers." In other words, there are always smarter people than you and your job as a leader is to find them or hire them, and then listen to them. In fact, within Lean Total Quality Management (TQM), not listening to your employees is one of the eight types of waste or "Muda" in an organization.

Fortunately for me, Doug took his own advice. After I launched the East Coast operations of Quantum in the late '80s and watched in dismay as HIV claimed the lives of two colleagues and countless hemophiliacs who tragically became infected with the virus, I suggested to Doug that Quantum develop a brand new segment of specialized services called disease management. I envisioned a service that would help patients with multiple conditions navigate our complex healthcare system with personalized health records and phone support from skilled care managers. Doug listened, then he politely said no. It wasn't right for Quantum, he said; primarily because it didn't fit its business model. However, knowing how passionate I was about the idea, he encouraged me to leave and start my own company, even helping me with initial funding.

That was the origin of Accordant Health Services, one of the nation's very first disease management companies. I launched Accordant from my home in 1994 with a generous severance from Quantum and the support of two well-known Silicon Valley venture capital firms. Despite their support, the first four years were a struggle. We were pushing an idea whose time had not yet come. Accordant brought patient education and information to the table, increasing quality and reducing costs for the most expensive diseases. Slowly, the managed care plans that we were selling to began to embrace this innovative model. Then everything seemed to really take off. By 2002, we engaged 200 nurses in our call center working directly with patients, gathering data the only way that was available then, from phone health risk assessments and insurance claims - the latter of which were quite dated compared to the near-real-time ambulatory data that we can consume today.

Accordant helped pioneer disease management in the US, driving recognition of the approach as a core strategy and capability for many healthcare organizations. But the way disease management worked – or in certain circumstances, failed to work - continued to bother me even after I sold the company to Advance PCS, now a part of CVS Caremark. Two thoughts in particular nagged at me, keeping me from moving on to other ventures.

First, because Accordant was in part distributed to patients through health plans, I knew physicians were sometimes suspicious of our motives. We had to work very hard to engage them. We did a good job, but I always felt that if we had done a better job of finding ways to engage physicians we could have had more impact on the industry and realized even better outcomes.

The second thought that troubled me was that we were never able to truly scale Accordant's business. Back then, the Internet was just beginning to go mainstream, there was no broadband to speak of, and we couldn't automate most of what Accordant was implementing. Moreover, having to depend on months-old claims data to deliver health coaching and interventions was less than ideal.

I spent the next few years thinking about these two problems and looking for solutions. Then a group of investors in Dallas approached me with the invitation to help lead Phytel. Phytel's future business model represented an opportunity to do what I had always hoped we could do at Accordant - leverage technology to automate patient engagement *and* collaborate with the providers to support the deployment of population health management for healthcare delivery.

At the time, Phytel's platform was focused on delivering automated outreach calls to address gaps in care, and appointment reminders to patients via the phone. But in it I saw the perfect platform on which to build automated solutions to support the entire care management process and to drive real patient engagement. Which is exactly what you need to do if you want to change patients' behaviors and make real improvements in health.

Not only did Phytel possess the perfect platform but the stars were aligning in terms of physician interest and incentives for quality and new technology. The industry was decisively shifting towards value-based pay-for-performance and the patient-centered medical home models, which are necessary components of successful population health management initiatives. Moreover, the federal government's incentives for electronic health record adoption were increasingly unleashing data that had previously been imprisoned on paper. Data was becoming the oxygen we needed to drive significant change in population health. With financial incentives for quality improvement combined with relevant digitized data, the sky would be the limit.

Eager to take advantage of the convergence of all these factors in the marketplace, we came up with a new product vision for Phytel:

- Motivate the patient to reconnect with their provider
- Optimize the all-too-infrequent encounter between provider and patient with tools, analytics, and alerts to improve the experience
- Extend the reach of physicians beyond the four walls of the practice with automated assessments, care management tools, reporting, and analytics

Our timing couldn't have been better. The opportunity before us – to deploy a population health management delivery model that can improve quality and bend the cost trend – is truly staggering. Virtually every element of health reform, from value-based reimbursement to accountable care organizations to the medical home, is based on the concept of managing populations of patients. Populations are the new denominator in the success equation. No longer are providers focused just on those patients who walk through the door. They're responsible for all their patients, no matter where they're being seen (or not seen).

All of which leads to the theme of this book. In the next five years I believe every provider in the top 50 metro areas in America will be required to execute a population health management strategy for a substantial portion of their patients. I call this "managing below the water line." Just as an iceberg hides most of its bulk below the surface, the greatest risk to providers' bottom lines is posed by the patients they *aren't* seeing and therefore aren't helping. Considering that 70 percent of today's high-cost patients were not in the high-cost category 12 months ago, in order to stay relevant in a value-based healthcare system, providers will need to be able to identify, stay in touch with, and improve the health of these patients – in other words, manage entire populations. With so much at stake, it's increasingly clear that you can no longer rely on manual methods to manage populations.

This book represents the culmination of efforts to date to help move the industry towards provider-led population health management. To the extent that it does that, the book will facilitate the transition of healthcare providers to a new way of patient-centered care delivery model, grounded on population health principles, and centered around the Triple Aim.

In the pages that follow you'll learn the key strategies employed by some of the nation's largest and most prestigious physician groups and health systems, which have employed automation to manage their populations and improve health outcomes. I hope and trust that you will find their experiences useful in your own journey to population health management.

Steve Schelhammer
Chief Executive Officer
Phytel, Inc.

Introduction

The $2.8-trillion health-care industry, as conventional wisdom has it, is a big ship to turn around. But employers, consumers, and government can no longer afford health-care costs that, while growing more slowly than in past years,[1] have reached stratospheric levels. The fee-for-service payment system that rewards providers for the volume of services has been implicated in the high cost of health care.[2] So, with a concerted push from payers, the industry is in the midst of a rapidly accelerating shift from fee-for-service to various forms of "pay for value."

The signs are all around us. In March 2014, Joseph R. Swedish, CEO of WellPoint, one of the nation's largest health insurers, said that WellPoint had tied a third of its commercial reimbursement to pay-for-value quality programs. By the end of the year, Swedish predicted, WellPoint "may have more than 50% of our commercial spend tied to value-based payments to providers."[3]

WellPoint's biggest competitor, UnitedHealth Group, is moving in the same direction. In February 2012, United said it was expanding its incentive programs, with a goal of offering at least half of its network physicians the ability to earn bonuses for value, quality, and efficiency within a few years.[4] Aetna has not made a similar prediction, but it is paying incentives to practices that have achieved recognition as patient-centered medical homes and is working with scores of provider groups and health systems to create accountable care organizations (ACOs).[5]

The Centers for Medicare and Medicaid Services (CMS) has also begun the transition to value-based payments. To start with, Medicare's Shared Savings Program (MSSP) is rewarding ACOs that create savings and meet quality goals.[6] While most of the 300-plus ACOs participating in this program are taking only upside risk today, many of them will have to take downside risk as well, starting in 2015, if they choose to renew their MSSP contracts.[7] CMS also has placed a small portion of hospitals' Medicare revenue at risk for achieving cost and quality goals, and it will begin applying the same program to physicians in 2015.[8,9]

What all of this means is that health-care providers can no longer avoid the reality that their current business models are obsolete. As they transition to the new care-delivery models, they must stop basing business decisions on how their clinicians and facilities can produce additional and ever-more-costly billable services. Those services used to be profit centers, but in the new world of value-based reimbursement, they are cost centers.

The fulcrum of profitability in this new world is maintaining or improving patients' health and delivering good outcomes. The only proven way to achieve those goals is to manage population health effectively and efficiently. To do that, health-care organizations need advanced health IT, including analytics and automation tools that enable them to transform their work processes.

Changing the mind-set

Except for group-model HMOs such as Kaiser Permanente and Group Health Cooperative, some large groups and individual practice associations (IPAs) in California, and a handful of health-care systems in other states, health-care providers are not well-positioned for population health management (PHM). While a number of health-care organizations are creating new structures designed for this purpose, the predominant mind-set in health-care is still oriented to fee-for-service "sick care." Physician practices still organize care around office visits, and hospitals focus on acute care within their four walls. The concept of caring for entire patient populations on a continuous basis, whether or not individual patients present for care, is only gradually seeping into the consciousness of healthcare managers and providers. And it is still difficult for some providers to accept the idea that filling beds and appointment slots is less important than ensuring that all patients receive recommended preventive and chronic care.

To transform themselves, organizations must reduce two kinds of waste: first, the avoidable tests, procedures, and hospital admissions and readmissions that lead to high costs for employers and consumers; and second, the internal waste that inflates the cost of care delivery. The reorganization of care processes can address both kinds of waste simultaneously by improving the quality and efficiency of care.

Organizations that go down this path need to adopt consistent policies and procedures, starting with a common set of clinical protocols. They have to form care teams that can coordinate care for every patient, tailoring their approach to the individual's health risks and conditions. They must restructure work flows so that each member of the care team is working up to the limit of his or her training and skill sets. And they must use their care managers as efficiently as possible so they can provide appropriate support to all patients who need help.

Electronic health records (EHRs), which have become widespread in the past few years, are essential to any population health management strategy. But EHRs are not designed to support PHM. While they can supply much of the data required to track and monitor patients' health and identify care gaps, they must be combined with claims data to provide a broad view of population health and to track individual patients across care settings. Moreover, providers need electronic registries to stratify their populations by health risk and to provide the near-real-time data required to intervene with subgroups of patients efficiently and in a timely manner.

The IT infrastructure for PHM must also include applications that automate the routine, repetitive work of care management. These automation tools offer several advantages. First, they can lower the cost of care management by taking over time-consuming chart research and outreach work. Second, they free up care managers to devote personal attention to high-risk patients who urgently need their help. Third, they allow providers to do pre-visit planning and post-visit follow-up on a consistent basis. Fourth, they can bring noncompliant patients back in touch with their personal physicians. And fifth, these tools enable organizations to quickly scale up their care-management efforts so they can continuously care for all of the patients in their population.

Most important, the combination of these tools offers a mechanism for engaging patients in their own health care. Without patient engagement, population health management is impossible.

Current trends

The rise of accountable care organizations (ACOs) in recent years reflects the concurrent emergence of value-based reimbursement and financial-risk contracts. Composed of physicians and hospitals that are committed to lowering costs and improving quality, ACOs must be able to deliver high-quality care within a budget. Strategies such as admitting patients to lower-cost hospitals and de-emphasizing expensive tests can help them do this in the short term; but in the long term, ACOs will have to manage population health well to be successful.

The patient-centered medical home (PCMH)—a holistic approach to primary care—is considered an essential building block of ACOs. The National Committee for Quality Assurance (NCQA) has given medical home recognition to more than 7,000 practices, comprised of about 30,000 providers, and the number of PCMHs is growing rapidly.[10]

The growth of patient-centered medical homes bodes well for the transformation of health care through ACOs. But to coordinate care effectively across care settings, the primary care physicians who have built medical homes must gain the cooperation of specialists, hospitals, and other health-care players in the medical neighborhood.

4

This might seem like a no-brainer at a time when health-care organizations are trying to prepare for value-based payments. But during this transitional period, when most specialists and hospitals still depend to a large extent on volume-based reimbursement, it's not easy for primary care doctors to persuade them that their future success depends on working with medical homes to coordinate care and reduce costs. Employed physicians will follow organizational directives to some extent, but at least half of physicians are still in independent practices.[11]

Some health-care organizations, including hospital systems and IPAs, have formed clinically integrated networks (CINs) that facilitate the collaboration of providers across care settings and business boundaries. These networks, which depend on health IT for communications and data sharing, can connect providers who otherwise might not collaborate with one another. Whether CINs will spread and help organize medical neighborhoods remains to be seen, but that's what they promise to do. If they succeed, they can provide the foundation of effective ACOs.

Patient engagement

As mentioned earlier, patient engagement is the sine qua non of population health management. At a population-wide level, this is about ensuring that patients take good care of themselves and comply with doctors' recommendations for proper preventive and chronic care and better health behavior. Fully half of disease prevention is up to patients, including their diet, exercise, and smoking behavior.[12]

But acute care, especially in hospitals and ambulatory surgery centers, also requires patient engagement for optimal outcomes. Not only must patients prepare for procedures, but they must also follow their post-discharge care plans and take the medications that have been prescribed for them.

It is unrealistic to expect some patients—especially those who are very ill, elderly, or poorly educated—to comply fully with their discharge instructions. Even if they want to, they may be unable to comply because they can't afford their medications or can't get an appointment with their primary care physician. So in a world of accountable care and value-based payments, providers must learn how to help these patients and get them involved in their own care after they leave the hospital.

The government's Meaningful Use EHR incentive program encourages providers to engage patients in several ways. In stage 2 of Meaningful Use, eligible professionals (EPs) and eligible hospitals must share records with patients online. EPs must also communicate with patients via secure online messaging and must send them reminders about preventive care.[13] The draft proposal for stage 3 recommends that providers be required to consider patient-generated data, such as health risk assessments and functional status surveys.[14]

Meanwhile, technology offers several other avenues for engaging patients. Automated patient outreach programs can message patients by e-mail, text, or phone, reminding them to make appointments with their doctor for needed preventive and chronic care.[15] Text messaging has been shown to help certain kinds of patients, such as people with diabetes and pregnant women, take better care of their health.[16] Educational materials tailored to individual patients can be made available online. And personal health records (PHRs), which can be used to download, store, and transmit health records, can help patients keep track of their care plans and medications and communicate with their providers.[17]

Recent advances in home telemonitoring and telehealth using mobile devices not only provide the opportunity for remote consultations, but also generate data that can keep providers and care managers apprised of patients' conditions between visits.[18] Of course, these new data streams could easily overwhelm providers; the information must be carefully screened so that caregivers see only relevant data.

A road map for population health management

No two health-care organizations are exactly the same or operate in the same environment with the same population. Nevertheless, as this book makes clear, provider organizations can follow a common road map that will take them close to where they want to go.

That map begins with the risk stratification of their population to identify which patients have the greatest health risks (and therefore, pose financial risks to the organization). Health-risk assessments administered to patients and analytics applied to clinical and claims data enable organizations to classify their populations.

Organizations should also reengineer their work processes, using Lean/ Six Sigma methods where possible, and then apply automation tools to make those processes more efficient.[19] The first step is to automate patient outreach, applying clinical protocols to registries that are either stand-alone or part of EHRs. These registries can be used to launch outbound messages to patients who have care gaps.

Another type of automation involves running reports on registry data to classify patients by subgroups. Care managers can then design campaigns to improve the health of specific subgroups, such as patients with type 2 diabetes and hypertension.

Many organizations make a mistake when they try to perform care management manually. They end up hiring a large number of nurses to scour medical records and call patients individually. This is not only a waste of time and money, but it also wastes the skills of these highly trained professionals.

Another common error is a failure to do pre-visit planning and post-visit follow-up. With the help of automation, it's relatively easy to find out what patients should do before office visits, such as getting tests done so that physicians can see the results. Similarly, tracking patient compliance after visits is not a big chore if the practice uses its EHR for automated tracking of orders for tests and referrals. Providers can find out whether patients filled prescriptions by getting online medication histories from Surescripts.[20]

With the encouragement of health plans, many providers are using claims data to identify their patients' care gaps and do predictive modeling. Claims data show all services that a plan member received from any provider, but they're frequently out-of-date and contain a lot of errors. Connecting a registry to EHR and billing data allows organizations to identify care gaps and high-risk patients in near-real time. Moreover, that actionable information can be supplied to providers at the point of care and to care managers as they plan their work and prioritize their cases. That allows them to intervene proactively with the patients who need help the most.

What this book is about

As the foregoing comments suggest, this book draws connections among the new care-delivery models, the components of population health management, and the types of health IT that are required to support those components. The key concept that ties all of this together is that PHM requires a high degree of automation to reach everyone in a population, engage those patients in self-care, and maximize the chance that they will receive the proper preventive, chronic, and acute care.

In the course of explaining how to do this, we also describe how health-care organizations are transforming themselves to manage population health and prepare for value-based reimbursement. The ACO, PCMH, and CIN models have already been discussed, and the advent of bundled payments will also have a major impact on hospital and post-acute care. But at its core, the transition to accountable care centers on care teams that take responsibility for managing and coordinating the services provided to individual patients. These care teams must also engage patients in caring for themselves and improving their health behavior. And as care teams become more sophisticated, many of them will use Lean thinking to continuously improve their own work processes.

The book is laid out in three sections, which progress from the general to the particular aspects of population health management. Section 1, entitled "New Delivery Models," first explains what PHM is and why it's important. Ensuing chapters cover ACOs and patient-centered medical homes, which are the favored vehicles for PHM.

Section 2, "How to Get There," discusses some fundamentals of the new delivery models, starting with the impact of Meaningful Use on the IT infrastructure that provider organizations must build to operationalize PHM. Other chapters in this section address clinical integration, predictive modeling applications, and the return on investment in IT solutions that help organizations take advantage of value-based payments.

Section 3, "Implementing Change," describes how organizations can use health IT to manage population health. This begins with the basics of care coordination and moves on to advanced methods of care management that utilize Lean thinking. Following a chapter on overall methods of patient engagement, we finish up with a discussion of post-discharge automation, which is another way to involve patients in their own care. Finally, in a brief concluding chapter, we suggest some next steps for organizations heading down the road to population health management.

While this book is intended for health-care executives and policy experts, anyone who is interested in health care can learn something from its exploration of the major issues that are stirring health care today. In the end, the momentous changes going on in health care will affect all of us.

Section I

New Delivery Models

Population Health Model

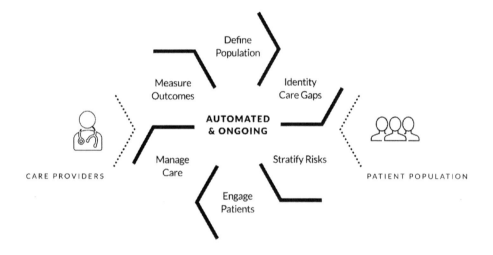

Chapter 1

Population Health Management

- *Introduction*: Health-care reform hasn't solved the major problems of our system with cost, quality, and access. To do that, we'll need to achieve the Triple Aim, including finding a way to manage population health efficiently.

- *Definition of PHM*: Population health management addresses the care of populations and the engagement of patients across care settings and over time. Above all, it requires an organized system of care.

- *Barriers to PHM*: In the United States, the biggest barriers to population health management are the fragmentation of care delivery, misaligned financial incentives, a lack of managed-care knowledge, and insufficient use of health information technology.

- *Beginnings of change*: Pay-for-performance and disease management have had little impact on population health improvement. But newer models such as patient-centered medical homes and accountable care organizations are more promising. The spread of EHRs also opens many new possibilities.

- *Crucial role of automation*: To have an impact on population health, health-care organizations must manage their entire patient populations. To do that effectively, they need electronic automation tools in addition to EHRs.

- *Three pillars of PHM*: Physicians should lead PHM, using three complementary approaches: strengthen and expand the doctor-patient relationship through the care team, reach out beyond the four walls of their offices, and optimize patient visits. Analytic and automation tools make this possible.

The protracted debate over health-care reform has highlighted the shortcomings of our health-care system. More than 8 million people have already been enrolled in private health plans through the state health insurance exchanges, and millions more have become eligible for Medicaid. But with the primary care workforce declining and a big increase in the demand for care anticipated, patient access to care is likely to shrink in the coming years.[1]

Quality is also an issue. The United States has a "sick care" system that is not designed to take good care of chronically ill patients, who generate about three quarters of health costs, or to prevent people from getting sick.[2] According to a famous RAND study, American adults receive recommended care only 55 percent of the time.[3] The gaps in treatment lead to unnecessary complications, ER visits, and hospitalizations—a major component of the waste in our system. So even if we had enough health-care providers, the rising costs of chronic-disease care would soon exceed our collective ability to pay for it.

The fragmentation of our delivery system and the poor communication among providers are prime reasons for the poor quality of care that many patients receive. For example, readmissions of patients with congestive heart failure have been on the rise for years. Today, about 20 percent of Medicare patients with CHF are readmitted within thirty days after discharge from the hospital. Some researchers have speculated that this may be related to shorter lengths of stay in the hospital.[4] But other studies show that better care management on the outpatient side could eliminate the majority of these readmissions.[5] In many cases, that care is not being provided because of poor handoffs from inpatient to outpatient care and lack of follow-up with the patients after discharge. In addition, there is no financial incentive for physicians to engage in the home care of patients, beyond the general supervision of home health nurses. In the case of heart failure, this continuous care is required to prevent emergencies that can lead to readmissions.

Except in a few large, integrated health-care systems and government systems that take financial responsibility for care, physicians are not generally paid to treat patients outside of office visits or to coordinate their care across care settings. Partly as a result, the continuity of care is disrupted at many points.[6]

At the same time, nonmedical determinants of health—which have a far greater impact on health than medical care—are not being properly addressed. Overeating, smoking, unsafe sex, lack of exercise, and other personal health behaviors are major components of health spending, yet physician counseling of patients is poorly reimbursed and usually confined to office visits for other problems. In addition, social determinants of health, such as access to care, health literacy, cultural barriers, income, and health insurance, affect the overall health of individuals and populations.

For these and many other reasons, the United States spends roughly twice as much on health care as other advanced countries do, yet the outcomes of our patients are inferior in many respects.[7] Health care is rapidly becoming unaffordable for many people, and both the federal and state governments are being bankrupted by skyrocketing medical costs.

Clearly, we need a radical change. We must reorganize the financing and the delivery of health care to provide greater value to both patients and society.

Myriad proposals have been made to restructure our system. One of the most promising is the "Triple Aim" of the Institute for Healthcare Improvement, formerly headed by Donald Berwick, MD, who first articulated this model. The Triple Aim program seeks to:

1) improve the experience of care,
2) improve the health of populations, and
3) reduce the per capita costs of care.[8]

This book will address the second aim: "improve the health of populations." We believe that by applying population health management principles, physicians and other providers can improve the health-care experience for patients while reducing cost growth to a manageable level.

What is population health management?

As Berwick and his colleagues point out in their paper on the Triple Aim, much of the current quality improvement efforts, such as "pay for performance" and Medicare's quality reporting programs, focus on single sites of care, including acute care hospitals and physician practices.[9] To really make a difference in outcomes, however, reformers must try to raise the quality of care and improve care coordination across all care settings. Also, this approach must be applied over a much longer period than that of a single episode of care.

These concepts lie at the core of population health management, which has been defined as a health-care approach focusing on "the health outcomes of individuals in a group and the distribution of outcomes in that group."[10] Former Kaiser Permanente CEO David Lawrence, MD, observes,

> Patients are just one of many such groups within a community. At any given time, most people do not worry about illness or wonder if they have one. They are not under treatment, and they see a physician infrequently. Yet for all people, lifestyles and behavior; race, culture, and language skills; and the environment in which they live are all important determinants of their individual health … Effective population health care includes interventions to moderate the impact of these powerful determinants [of health].[11]

Key components

So population health management, or PHM as we will hereafter refer to it, addresses not only longitudinal care across the continuum of care, but also personal health behaviors that may contribute to or prevent healing or disease. Based on the experience of Kaiser Permanente and other organizations that are dedicated to PHM,[12] here are some of the other aspects of this approach to care:

- *An organized system of care.* Health-care providers must be organized, even if they're only electronically linked and have agreed to follow certain clinical protocols to improve the quality of care.
- *Care teams.* Physicians and other clinicians work in care teams to provide multiple levels of patient care and education on a consistent basis.
- *Coordination across care settings.* Patients have a personal physician who coordinates their care and guides them through the system.
- *Access to primary care.* Primary care is vitally necessary to make sure patients receive necessary preventive, chronic, and acute care.
- *Centralized resource planning.* Resources are allocated to make sure that individual patients receive all necessary care and that available resources are optimally applied across the population.
- *Continuous care.* Providers are available to patients both during and between office visits, and all forms of communication, including secure electronic messaging, are appropriately utilized.
- *Patient self-management education.* With the help of printed and online materials, care teams help patients learn how to manage their own conditions to the extent possible.
- *Focus on health behavior/lifestyle changes.* Providers and the educational materials they offer reinforce the need for healthy lifestyles across the population.
- *Interoperable electronic health records.* EHRs are used to store and retrieve data, not only on individual patients, but on the status of the population. They are also used to track orders, referrals, and other care processes to ensure that patients receive the care they need. And by exchanging data with other clinical systems, interoperable EHRs provide physicians with information that helps them make better decisions.

- *Electronic registries.* Whether or not registries are part of EHRs, they are important components of PHM, because they enable caregivers to track and manage all of the services provided to or due for their patient population, as well as subgroups of that population.

In addition, shared decision making has become an important tool in population health management. This includes providing and explaining information to patients about treatment options to help them make informed decisions about their care.

Until recently, major components of PHM were found mainly in group-model HMOs like Kaiser Permanente and Group Health Cooperative of Puget Sound; large integrated delivery systems like Intermountain Healthcare, Geisinger Clinic, and the Henry Ford Health System; and the Veterans Affairs health system and the Military Health System. But accountable care organizations, the Medicare Shared Savings Program, and commercial risk contracts are all increasing interest in PHM among other organizations as well.

Obstacles to PHM

In the United States, the biggest barriers to population health management are the fragmentation of care delivery, perverse financial incentives, a lack of managed-care knowledge, and insufficient use of health information technology.

According to the Institute of Medicine's 2001 report *Crossing the Quality Chasm*, "The current health care delivery system is highly decentralized ... In a population increasingly afflicted by chronic conditions, the health care delivery system is poorly organized to provide care to those with such conditions ... The challenge before us is to move from today's highly decentralized, cottage industry to one that is capable of providing primary and preventive care, caring for the chronically ill, and coping with acute and catastrophic services."[13]

The fee-for-service reimbursement system is the opposite of the payment approach that is suited to PHM. Fee-for-service incentivizes physicians to perform more services, rather than help patients get well or prevent them from getting sick. Because third-party payers usually pay doctors only for services performed in their offices, the hospital, or some other institutional setting, physicians have no incentive to communicate with patients online or on the phone or care for them at home. There are perverse incentives in other payment approaches, including capitation, which motivates doctors to do as little for patients as possible, and straight salary, which doesn't encourage them to work hard.[14] A new payment approach is needed for PHM.

Managing within a budget

Because most physicians are used to practicing in the fee-for-service system, they have traditionally not had to manage care within a budget.[15] (Budgeting is part of the central resource planning referred to above.) Since there are limits to the available health-care resources, physicians must learn how to order tests and perform procedures more appropriately, consistent with evidence-based guidelines. Many doctors will object that they must practice defensive medicine to guard against malpractice suits. Because physicians are so concerned about this, malpractice reform could help accelerate the evolution of PHM.

Finally, the health-care industry needs to make much better use of information technology and improve the quality of data in the system if PHM is going to become a reality. This includes not only EHRs and health information exchanges, but also registries and applications that use clinical protocols and sophisticated algorithms to identify individuals with care gaps and to trigger communications to those patients and their physicians.[16]

The government's Meaningful Use incentive program has helped boost the adoption of EHRs, which are now used by 61 percent of physician practices.[17] Most physicians are still not using EHRs for quality improvement or for tracking patient health between office visits. However, Meaningful Use, particularly the stage 2 and the proposed stage 3 criteria, encourage physicians to take advantage of EHRs and other kinds of certified applications to manage population health.

Beginnings of change

Over the past fifteen or twenty years, approaches such as pay for performance and disease management have had a very limited effect on quality improvement. Pay-for-performance programs focus on a relatively small set of measures, confuse physicians with conflicting goals from multiple health plans, don't reward improvement, and often use sample sizes that are too small to show how well individual physicians are doing on particular metrics.[18]

Disease management, a systematic approach to caring for patients with chronic diseases, has taken two different forms. The chronic-care model, a method of integrating all of the care for particular chronic conditions across providers and over time,[19] requires the resources of a large organization, such as a group-model HMO, and cannot be readily applied in small practices, although they can undertake parts of it.[20] The insurance-based model of disease management tries to overcome the fragmentation of the market by taking a more patient-focused approach. The insurers and third-party disease management firms rely on nurse care managers, who telephonically interact with patients to educate them about their condition and their health risks and work with them over time to effect behavior change. The major flaw in this model is that physicians are involved in the process only peripherally, if at all.

More promising models have emerged in the past few years. These include the patient-centered medical home (PCMH) and the accountable care organization (ACO).

The PCMH is designed to help primary care practices of all sizes provide comprehensive primary care. Among its key components are a personal physician who is responsible for all of a patient's ongoing care; team care; a whole-person orientation; care coordination facilitated by the use of health IT; a care-planning process based on a robust partnership between physicians and patients; and enhanced access to care, including non-visit care.[21]

While thousands of practices have been recognized as patient-centered medical homes, practices that try to become medical homes encounter some significant obstacles. First, small primary care practices may lack the time and the resources to transform themselves and acquire the necessary information technology[22]; second, they may find it difficult to gain the cooperation of specialists and hospitals; and third, most physicians do not receive adequate financial support from payers for coordinating care.[23] However, a growing number of health plans are paying care-coordination fees to primary care practices that are recognized as medical homes.

Accountable care organizations consist of hospitals and physicians that take collective responsibility for the cost and quality of care for all patients in their population. While related in some respects to the original HMO concept, the ACO grew out of the ideas of Elliott Fisher, a professor at Dartmouth Medical School, CMS Administrator Donald Berwick, and Commonwealth Fund President Karen Davis.[24] It is complementary to the PCMH in the sense that it could enable primary care physicians to benefit financially from improving care coordination. ACOs cannot function without a strong foundation of primary care.[25]

ACOs may be single business entities, such as a group-model HMO or an integrated delivery system. But they could also involve an "extended medical staff" or a contracting network that includes a health-care system. IPAs that have evolved into clinically integrated organizations could also serve as ACOs.

Partly because of the Medicare Shared Savings Program (MSSP), ACOs have grown rapidly in recent years, and there are now more than 500 ACOs.[26] Many health-care organizations are forming ACOs to participate in the MSSP and/or commercial risk and shared-savings contracts.

The widespread development of ACOs, perhaps with medical homes at their core, would provide a powerful impetus for a shift from the current care-delivery model to PHM. With the backing of large organizations and the introduction of financial incentives that encourage an outcomes-oriented, patient-centered care model, PHM could become the dominant model of health care.

The crucial role of automation

Some observers have raised serious objections to this rosy scenario. Consultant and health-care expert Jeff Goldsmith, for example, points out that the effort of insurance companies to pass financial risk to providers proved to be the Achilles heel of managed care in the 1990s.[27] This doesn't necessarily doom ACOs, however, because they will have to be accountable for quality as well as for cost. This should prevent a public backlash similar to the one that defeated HMOs. In addition, information technology has advanced to the point where all patients in a population can be identified, risk-stratified, and provided with advanced self-management tools to prevent exacerbation of their illnesses. Physicians didn't have these tools in the heyday of HMOs.

David Lawrence, the former CEO of Kaiser Permanente, points to another problem: the difficulty that primary care physicians would have in making the transition to the new delivery model. (While he cites this difficulty in regard to the medical home, the same criticism could be applied to ACOs, because primary care physicians are the linchpins of care coordination in both models.) Lawrence believes that to increase access to primary care, we need to make use of "disruptive innovations," including retail clinics, employer-based wellness programs, home telemonitoring of patients with chronic conditions, and new methods of educating patients in self-management.[28]

Manage the entire population

To be able to manage all aspects of health from wellness to complex care, health-care organizations must assess the entire population, taking advantage of online or web-based programs. Patients can then be stratified into various stages across the spectrum of health. Those who are well need to stay well by getting preventive tests completed; those who have health risks need to change their health behaviors so they don't develop the conditions they're at risk for; and those who have chronic conditions need to prevent further complications by closing care gaps and also working on health behaviors. Technology can be very helpful in assessing and stratifying patients and targeting interventions to the right people. The automation of the processes provides a more efficient and effective way to do population health management.

What's really needed for successful PHM is an electronic infrastructure that performs much of the routine, time- and labor-intensive work in the background for physicians and their staffs. Fortunately, most of the tools for building such an infrastructure already exist, although they tend to be scattered and underused. When these tools are pulled together and applied in a coordinated, focused manner, they will be a powerful force for change.

Technology is not a substitute for the physician-patient relationship, which is the basis of continuous care. In fact, physicians and their care teams can have a major, positive effect on patient experience, compliance, and behavior change. But to the extent that automation tools are used to strengthen that relationship and enable physicians and care teams to provide value-added services that help patients improve their health proactively, these technologies can help drive population health management.[29]

Three Pillars of PHM

To do PHM properly, physicians and their care teams must strengthen their relationships with patients in a variety of ways, including making sure that they come in for needed preventive and chronic care. Care teams, which include physicians, midlevel practitioners, medical assistants, social workers, and nurse educators, must optimize the services they provide to patients during office visits. And they must extend their reach beyond the four walls of their offices to provide a continuous healing relationship. The appropriate IT tools can facilitate achievement of all three goals, while lessening the burden on practices.

One of the best ways to strengthen the doctor-patient relationship is to combine an electronic registry with an automated method of communicating with patients who are overdue for preventive or chronic-care services. The patient demographic and clinical data in the registry can come from billing systems or electronic health records, as well as labs and pharmacies. The registry provides lists of patients with particular health conditions and shows what has been done for them and when. By continuously running evidence-based clinical protocols and a communications engine, the registry can trigger outbound calls or secure online messages to patients who need to make an appointment with their doctor for particular services at specific intervals.

Besides improving the health of the population, this automated messaging also brings patients back in touch with their physicians—in some cases, after long intervals of noncontact. Without requiring any effort from the doctors or their staff, this combination of tools enhances the doctor-patient relationship and helps to close gaps in care, while also increasing practice revenues as a byproduct.

Optimization of visits requires preparation by both the patient and the care team. The first thing patients should do is fill out a health risk assessment (HRA), either online or in the office, that shows the state of their health and what they're doing about it. The patients should also receive educational materials, including online multimedia tools, to prepare them for the office visit.

Physicians and other care-team members need actionable, patient-specific reports that combine data from their EHRs with data from registries, other providers, and HRAs to show what has been done for the patient, the gaps in their care that need to be filled, and nonmedical issues that may be impeding patients' abilities to manage their health and health risks. Care teams also require population-level reports that can help them figure out how to improve the quality of care. While advanced EHRs include health maintenance alerts, they may lack clinical dashboards that present key markers of the patient's status, may be unable to compile data across a patient population to support quality improvement, and may be unsuited for patient care by a multidisciplinary care team.[30]

What's needed is a sophisticated rules engine that can incorporate disparate types of data with evidence-based guidelines, generating reports that provide many different views of the information. For example, the entire patient population could be filtered by payer, activity center, provider, health condition, and care gaps. The same filters could be applied to patients with a particular condition, such as diabetes, to find out where the practice needs to improve its diabetes care.

The same approach could be used to produce reports for care teams at the point of care. For a diabetic patient, a report related to that condition would show the patient's blood pressure and body-mass index, whether he or she had had an HbA1c test within a certain period of time, and his or her HbA1c level, among other data points. If the reports were combined with the registry and the patient messaging software, the physician or midlevel practitioner would be able find out whether and when the patient had been contacted to come in for an office visit or get a test done and whether he or she had made an appointment. In addition, the care team can use these reports to reach out to patients who need educational materials or one-on-one educational and goal-setting sessions to learn how to manage their conditions.

Extending the reach of the care team beyond the office requires both the willingness of providers to stay in touch with the patient and modalities that help patients care for themselves. Automation can help both sides achieve those goals without excessive effort. For example, when patients fill out an HRA, they could receive educational materials tailored to their conditions, and they could be directed to appropriate self-help programs for, say, smoking cessation or losing weight. And if physicians had automated methods to contact patients and remind them of what they need to do to improve their health, the practice would be more likely to perform that component of PHM.

Conclusion

To create a sustainable health-care system that provides affordable, high-quality health care to all, we will have to adopt a population health management approach. While the transition to PHM will be difficult for providers and patients alike, the change could be facilitated and accelerated through the use of health information technology, self-management tools, and automated reminders that are persistent in changing behaviors.

The current generation of EHRs lacks many of the features required to improve population health. But by combining EHRs with adjunctive technologies that already exist, physicians can rapidly move to PHM strategies that will benefit all of their patients and enhance the physician-patient relationship.

These new technologies are important to the new accountable care organizations (ACOs) that are sprouting everywhere. The next chapter describes the kind of IT infrastructure that ACOs need to do population health management.

Chapter 2

Accountable Care Organizations

- *Introduction*: The Affordable Care Act authorized a Medicare shared-savings program for accountable care organizations, and private payers are also contracting with ACOs. To succeed, ACOs must learn how to manage population health effectively.

- *The ACO environment*: Physicians and hospitals, which are competing for leadership of ACOs, must find ways to share revenue equitably within these organizations. While payers don't want to push risk on providers too rapidly, some advanced ACOs have already accepted global capitation contracts.

- *Group practice demonstration*: Medicare's Physician Group Practice demonstration, a precursor of the ACO shared-savings program, offers some lessons about how large groups can approach this reimbursement method. The results show that it was easier for the participating groups to improve quality than to generate shared savings.

- *Population health management*: ACOs have strong incentives to improve population health to meet quality goals and reduce costs. To do that, they must stress non-visit care and disease management, build care teams, and work with patients to improve their health behavior.

- *Role of information technology*: Population health management requires clinical integration, which cannot exist without a robust IT infrastructure. In addition, a range of automation tools are needed for cost-effective care management and outreach to patients. When coupled with care transformation services, information technology is most effective for scaling the reach of the care team across the ACO cohort(s) and lays the foundation for managing population health.

The Patient Protection and Affordable Care Act (PPACA) of 2010 focuses mainly on regulating health insurance and expanding coverage. But the legislation also addresses the role of the health-care delivery system in health spending growth.

In this area, the law's major thrust is to change how providers are paid. Among the approaches that Congress authorized the government to undertake is one that involves "accountable care organizations" (ACOs), which are health-care provider groups that are designed to be accountable for the cost and quality of care.

Specifically, the PPACA authorized the Centers for Medicare and Medicaid Services (CMS) to launch a shared-savings program with ACOs in 2012. Under this approach, an ACO that meets specified quality goals can split with CMS any savings that surpass a minimum level.[1]

ACOs that participate in the Medicare Shared Savings Program must consist of providers that "work together to manage and coordinate care for Medicare fee-for-service beneficiaries." Among the ACOs in the MSSP are organizations based on individual practice networks, group practices, partnerships of hospitals and physicians, hospitals and their employed doctors, and federally qualified health centers. ACOs must meet thresholds on thirty-three quality measures and save more than a minimum amount to qualify for payments equal to 50 percent of the amount they save CMS above a benchmark related to their historical performance. A few ACOs have elected to take downside risk as well, in return for a higher percentage of savings.[2]

The Medicare Shared-Savings Program, which is not a pilot, potentially affects all patients covered by traditional Medicare. As a result, the ACO provision has generated strong interest among group practices and health-care organizations.

The ACO initiatives of some commercial insurers are also attracting attention from providers. Some of the private ACO contracts involve financial risk,[3] and others are limited to gainsharing. But the majority of the 600 current ACOs are involved in the MSSP and other CMS programs.[4,5]

In the first year of the MSSP, fifty-four of the 114 participants that joined the program in 2012 had total costs that fell below their budget benchmarks, but only twenty-nine reduced spending enough to qualify for a total of $126 million in shared savings. The other sixty ACOs generated costs above their benchmarks.[6]

Other new reimbursement methods

The ACO concept dovetails with other new reimbursement methods that payers are piloting, including payment bundling and patient-centered medical homes. Further down the road, it's likely that shared savings will transition to some type of payment bundling and, eventually, global capitation (a fixed payment for all care provided to each patient). But right now, the government and private insurers are proceeding with caution, because they know that the vast majority of providers are not ready to assume that much financial risk. Moreover, there are questions about how much limitation on provider choice the public is willing to accept.

Whichever direction the reimbursement changes take, they will require providers to do population health management (PHM). In the case of ACOs, the reasons are transparent: these organizations must manage the full spectrum of care and must be accountable for a defined patient population.[7] Unless an ACO is capable of tracking the health status of and the care provided to every one of its patients, it is unlikely to produce significant savings or meet the quality benchmarks of CMS. And when organizations take on financial risk, it is absolutely essential for them to learn how to prevent illness and manage care as well as possible. The more risk that providers assume, the better they have to be at managing their populations' health.

The ACO environment

A growing number of health-care organizations have partnered with health plans to implement ACOs.[8] While most insurance companies are still reluctant to offer global capitation contracts, they see opportunities in working with ACOs to lower costs and improve quality.

Meanwhile, hospitals and doctors that are partnered in ACOs must find ways to share revenue. But gainsharing between hospitals and physicians is still fairly uncommon, having only recently emerged from a regulatory deep freeze.[9] In addition, health policy expert Jeff Goldsmith points out,[10] hospitals and independent physicians have moved further apart in recent years as medical and surgical specialists have pulled more services out of the hospital into their offices, imaging centers, and ambulatory surgery centers.

Other trends are moving in the opposite direction. Hospitals are employing more and more physicians, including specialists.[11] They are doing so partly for competitive reasons and partly because they believe that they will need to have physicians' cooperation when reimbursement methods change.

The Federal Trade Commission, meanwhile, has given a handful of IPAs and physician-hospital organizations (PHOs) approval to negotiate insurance contracts because they are clinically integrated and are therefore able to improve the quality of care.[12] Many health-care systems are moving toward clinical integration with their physicians, whether or not the latter are employed. And the spread of health-care information technology is expected to accelerate this process.[13]

Snapshot of current ACOs

Currently, the biggest private-sector ACO experiment is the "alternative quality contract" of Massachusetts Blue Cross and Blue Shield.[14] This is actually a global capitation agreement, with two features that differentiate it from the old HMO risk contracts: first, participants can qualify for graduated quality incentives, and second, the insurer pledges not to reduce their budgets in future years. In return, the contract holders promise to gradually cut cost growth to the rate of inflation.

Sixteen organizations currently participate in the Massachusetts Blues' alternative quality contract. They range in size from Partners Healthcare in Boston to the physician-hospital organization of Lowell General Hospital in Lowell, Massachusetts.[15]

Other organizations that have formed ACOs include the Greater Rochester (NY) IPA, Advocate Health Care in Chicago, Brown & Toland in San Francisco, Hill Physicians in San Ramon, Calif., and Healthcare Partners in Los Angeles.

Hill Physicians is participating in a three-way pilot involving Dignity Health and Blue Shield of California.[16] That pilot, funded by the California Public Employees Retirement System, is focused on reducing HMO costs by sharing financial risk.

Healthcare Partners, a multistate physician group and IPA based in Los Angeles, is engaged in another ACO pilot with Anthem Blue Cross. This pilot started with a shared-savings approach in the first year, but was expected to graduate to global capitation over the five-year contract period.[17]

The Anthem-Healthcare Partners venture is one of several pilots being conducted across the country under the aegis of the Engelberg Center for Health Care Reform at the Brookings Institution and the Dartmouth Institute for Health Policy and Clinical Practice. The leaders of those research organizations—Mark McClellan, MD, and Elliott Fisher, MD, respectively—are among the founders of the ACO movement. They formed the Brookings-Dartmouth ACO Learning Network to promote the concept to health-care organizations.[18]

Some observers question whether ACOs can succeed in most areas unless hospitals take the lead in organizing them. Yet there is nothing in the CMS regulations that requires hospitals to lead or even be a direct participant in ACOs. The only requirements are that ACOs include primary care physicians and serve at least 5,000 Medicare patients each.[19] But because an ACO must coordinate care across all care settings, it must secure the cooperation of one or more hospitals. So, while both physician organizations and hospitals would prefer to be in charge, they will have to learn how to work together.

Other experts doubt that a shared-savings program that offers only rewards without risk will get physicians' attention and motivate them to change how they practice. They also wonder how patients will react to the idea of having a personal physician coordinate all of their care, when the patients are used to going to any physician they want to see. These observers view the Medicare approach as a first step toward partial or full capitation of health-care organizations.[20]

Group practice demonstration

These are valid points, but the history of Medicare's Physician Group Practice (PGP) demonstration—an important precursor of the shared-savings program—offers some reasons to hope that large provider groups will be able to use CMS's shared-savings approach in constructive ways.

The PGP pilot, which involved ten large groups and health-care systems, began in 2005 and ended in March 2010. CMS paid the participants up to 80 percent of Medicare's savings from inpatient and outpatient care in excess of 2 percent of historical costs. Half of the bonuses were based on efficiency, and the other half came from meeting quality targets.

Over the five years of the PGP demonstration, the groups did well on CMS's quality measures. In the fifth year, seven groups achieved benchmark-level performance on all thirty-two measures, and the other groups did so on at least thirty measures. In addition, the PGPs increased their quality scores on diabetes, heart-failure, and cancer-screening measures by at least 9 percentage points over the five years.

However, only half of the PGP participants were able to exceed a 2 percent savings threshold after three years. The Marshfield Clinic alone earned about half of the total savings, and four other groups accounted for most of the rest.[21]

Each participant used different techniques to improve care and reduce costs. For example, the Dartmouth-Hitchcock Clinic in Bedford, New Hampshire, focused on the use of electronic registries and patient education. The Everett Clinic, a large multispecialty group in Washington state, concentrated on improving primary care and radiology services, as well as the handoffs between inpatient and outpatient care settings. But all of the participants, in their own ways, were trying to upgrade their ability to manage population health.

The Everett Clinic netted some of the shared savings in the second year of the pilot, but none in the third year. The group successfully reduced the cost of imaging services and improved its understanding of how to manage high-cost subpopulations who need complex care. But the clinic also encountered some significant obstacles, including difficulty in correlating health risk scores with cost-effectiveness, the retrospective nature of the model, problems in getting providers outside the group to cooperate, and difficulty in persuading patients to use their primary care physician as a care coordinator.[22]

Population health management

US health care costs much more per capita than the systems of other advanced countries but does not deliver better results.[23] The reasons are well-known: The United States has a fragmented, chaotic care delivery system, health-care providers are incentivized to provide high service volume rather than high-quality care, we have too few primary care physicians and too many specialists, and our system is provider-centered rather than patient-centered.[24]

To turn this bloated, wasteful health-care system around, policy makers and health-policy experts are focusing on population health management

(PHM). As discussed in chapter 1, PHM has been defined as a health-care approach that emphasizes "the health outcomes of individuals in a group and the distribution of outcomes in that group." It addresses not only longitudinal care across the continuum of care, but also personal health behavior that may contribute to the evolution or exacerbation of diseases.[25]

Among the key characteristics of health organizations that conduct PHM are an organized system of care; the use of multidisciplinary care teams; coordination across care settings; enhanced access to primary care; centralized resource planning; continuous care, both in and outside of office visits; patient self-management education; a focus on health behavior and lifestyle changes; the use of interoperable electronic health records; and the use of registries and other tools essential to the automation of PHM.[26]

Today, as mentioned earlier, the main practitioners of PHM are group-model HMOs, large integrated delivery systems, the Veterans Affairs health system, and the Military Health System. But as ACOs gain traction, the providers that belong to them are increasingly trying to manage population health, too.

Whether the financial incentive is shared savings or global budgets, ACOs have a strong motive to maintain health, prevent disease, and control chronic conditions so that they don't lead to ER visits and hospitalizations. To achieve these goals, ACOs have to stress non-visit care and disease management, including home monitoring of the sickest patients. They have to build care teams that are capable of tracking patients' health status and ensuring that they receive recommended care. And they have to incentivize providers to work with patients to improve their health behavior and their compliance with care plans.

ACOs share many of these objectives with patient-centered medical homes. For example, a physician whose practice serves as a medical home must coordinate care, improve patient self-management skills, track the services provided to patients, and maintain contact with patients between visits. Medical homes also use electronic tools such as EHRs and registries.[27] The primary care practices that serve as medical homes are generally much smaller than ACOs and may lack the ability to induce specialists and hospitals to cooperate with them.[28] Nevertheless, a practice that qualifies as a medical home has gone a long way toward being able to function within an ACO.

An effective ACO must not only take excellent care of patients who present for care, but must also try to monitor and stay in contact with people who do not have contact, or rarely have contact, with health-care providers. The importance of communicating with this segment of the population is profound, because it includes many individuals who are or will become sick and need acute or chronic care at some point in time. Therefore, an ACO that proactively addresses the health needs of this cohort will be able to control costs better than one that doesn't.

Role of information technology

To be successful, an ACO must be clinically integrated, which means that physicians and other providers must communicate and exchange key clinical information with each other. Until recently, this was very difficult, because most clinical data were locked up in paper files that were inaccessible to providers outside of a particular hospital or practice. Even the delivery of lab results was still done mostly by fax, courier, or mail. Now, as EHRs become widespread because of the government's Meaningful Use incentive program, all of this is starting to change. In addition, care transformation services that help integrate information technology into daily work flow can be effective at driving clinical integration and population health management.

EHRs are crucial to clinical integration. Not only can they make it easier for caregivers to document and retrieve patient data, but they also hold the key to health information exchange with other providers—if they ever become interoperable.

Despite the enormous increase in the amount of digitized health information, however, most EHRs are still incapable of exchanging structured data. The clinical summaries that certified EHRs must be able to exchange in Meaningful Use stage 2 use a specially formatted document known as the consolidated CDA (C-CDA). EHRs from different vendors can exchange these summaries, but the data in them cannot flow into the data fields in electronic charts.

The federal government has spent more than half a billion dollars to help states develop health information exchanges (HIEs). While it's not clear that this effort has substantially improved the ability of providers to exchange patient data, a recent report shows that in 2013, more than six in ten hospitals exchanged health information with outside providers—a 51 percent increase since 2008. Fifty seven percent of hospitals exchanged data with ambulatory providers outside of their system—although only about a quarter of hospitals notified outside primary care providers when their patients entered one of the hospitals' ERs.[29]

Meanwhile, as the federal grants expire, regional HIEs are still searching for a business model,[30] and an increasing number of health-care organizations are building private exchanges.[31] Clinician-to-clinician messaging using the Direct secure-messaging protocol is also growing as the Direct infrastructure evolves.[32]

Automation tools

EHRs have some drawbacks as tools for performing population health management. They are not designed for tracking populations, providing actionable reports on care gaps, or sending alerts to patients.[33] ACOs will need not only EHRs, but also supplemental technologies that automate the work of monitoring, educating, and maintaining contact with the patient population.

These tools, which should be used in conjunction with EHRs, include electronic registries, multiple outreach and communications methods, software that can stratify a population by health status, and health risk assessment programs that trigger alerts and provide educational materials to patients. Automated PHM tools ensure that the routine, repetitive work of managing population health is done in the background, freeing up doctors and nurses to do the work that only they can do.

For example, registries can be programmed to generate reports on the care gaps of patients for care coordinators and care managers in practices. The care managers can use the information to prepare care teams for patient visits and to ensure that patients are receiving recommended services across the continuum of care. By automating patient communications, registries combined with outreach tools also make it easy to send alerts to every patient who needs to be seen for follow-up.

These supplemental technologies can also aid ACOs in managing population health at the macro level. A sophisticated rules engine can integrate disparate types of data with evidence-based guidelines, generating reports that provide many different views of the information. For example, the entire patient population could be filtered by payer, activity center, provider, health condition, and care gaps. The same filters could be applied to all patients with a particular condition to find out where the ACO needs to improve its care for that disease.

ACO management could also use this type of information to pinpoint where the coordination of care is breaking down. For example, if an unusual number of patients with a particular condition were being readmitted to the hospital, that might indicate a problem with outpatient follow-up.

Another important determinant of population health is the degree to which patients are coached on improving their health behavior. Automation tools can also help in this area. For example, when a patient fills out a health risk assessment online or in a practice computer kiosk, that patient can receive educational materials tailored to his or her condition and can be directed to appropriate self-help programs for, say, smoking cessation or losing weight.

Conclusion

Largely because of the health-care reform law's authorization of a Medicare shared-savings program, accountable care organizations (ACOs) are generating excitement among health-care providers. If ACOs become widespread, they could become a powerful force for establishing population health management as the primary approach to quality improvement and cost containment in the United States.

To do PHM properly, ACOs must use a range of information technologies. These include not only electronic health records, but also supplemental applications that automate the routine work of tracking, educating, and communicating with patients. These tools make it possible to do PHM comprehensively and cost-effectively, allowing ACO members to benefit economically from shared-savings, bundled-payment, and global-capitation programs.

Many health-care organizations are setting up ACOs. But only the ACOs that achieve clinical integration and learn how to do population health management will succeed. Therefore, information technologies, including automation tools, are essential components of ACO success.

Patient-centered medical homes (PCMHs), often considered the building blocks of ACOs, also need EHRs and other health IT tools to perform their primary task of care coordination. The next chapter explains what medical homes are and why health IT is essential to their mission.

Population Health within the Medical Neighborhood

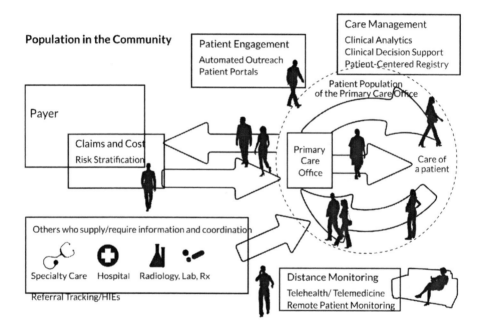

Population in the Community

Patient Engagement
Automated Outreach
Patient Portals

Care Management
Clinical Analytics
Clinical Decision Support
Patient-Centered Registry

Patient Population
of the Primary Care Office

Payer

Claims and Cost
Risk Stratification

Primary
Care
Office

Care of
a patient

Others who supply/require information and coordination

Specialty Care   Hospital   Radiology, Lab, Rx

Referral Tracking/HIEs

Distance Monitoring
Telehealth/ Telemedicine
Remote Patient Monitoring

Chapter 3

Patient-Centered Medical Homes

- *Introduction*: The patient-centered medical home movement is growing rapidly, with support from both private insurers and the government. But medical homes can't achieve their full potential until they can integrate with the medical neighborhood and start automating care management.
- *PCMH background*: The PCMH model is essentially holistic primary care, in which physician-led care teams coordinate and manage care. The new 2014 criteria for PCMH recognition from the National Committee for Quality Assurance (NCQA) continue to emphasize health IT and mirror some of the requirements of Meaningful Use stage 2.
- *Challenges and solutions*: Primary care practices must completely reengineer themselves to become patient-centered medical homes. While small practices can do much of this, even large multispecialty groups lack many of the requisite components of the PCMH. The cost of creating and maintaining a medical home could be much lower if PCMH functions in the practices are highly automated.
- *Role of information technology*: EHRs are necessary but not sufficient for practices that aim to become PCMHs. They have some of the necessary tools, but fall short in the area of population health management. External registries and automation tools can fill the gap.

Because of the current national focus on accountable care organizations (ACOs), attention has shifted away from the patient-centered medical home (PCMH), an approach designed to rebuild primary care and improve care coordination. Nevertheless, the PCMH model is continuing to grow rapidly and to attract support from providers, payers, and consumer groups.

According to a survey by the Medical Group Management Association (MGMA), 70 percent of primary care physicians and nonphysician providers are transforming their practices into patient-centered medical homes or are interested in doing so. Twenty percent of the respondents said they'd already been accredited or recognized as a PCMH.[1]

The National Committee for Quality Assurance (NCQA) has recognized 10 percent of US primary care practices—nearly 7,000 sites—as patient-centered medical homes.[2]

The Joint Commission, URAC, and some Blue Cross and Blue Shield plans have given their PCMH stamps of approval to additional practices.

Many payers support the medical home movement. The NCQA website lists three dozen health plans that use NCQA recognition in their PCMH incentive programs.[3] Some plans, like Aetna and Cigna, require this recognition for practices to participate in their high-performance networks.[4]

Altogether, more than ninety commercial health insurers have embraced the PCMH approach, according to the Patient-Centered Primary Care Collaborative (PCPCC). These include such major carriers as WellPoint, Aetna, Humana, and United. More than 4 million Blue Cross Blue Shield members in thirty-nine states are participating in some type of PCMH initiative.[5]

The Centers for Medicare and Medicaid Services (CMS) is participating in multi-payer PCMH projects in eight states.[6] At the same time, forty-two state Medicaid programs are involved in PCMH demonstrations.[7] And the Veterans Health Administration is in the midst of a three-year program to build patient-centered medical homes in more than 900 primary care clinics.[8]

Initial results are promising

Early evidence shows that the patient-centered medical home can improve access to high-quality care and the management of chronic conditions. For example, one study of care provided under PCMH principles found patients with diabetes had significant reductions in cardiovascular risk, patients with congestive heart failure had 35 percent fewer hospital days, and asthma and diabetes patients were more likely to receive appropriate therapy.[9]

A study of seven PCMH demonstration projects reported that the strategy resulted in reductions in ER visits ranging from 15 percent to 50 percent, and decreases in hospital admissions ranging from 10 percent to 40 percent.[10] Another paper, based on the experience of Group Health Cooperative, a large integrated delivery system, showed that the PCMH model increased patient satisfaction and staff morale and improved quality without raising costs.[11]

In fact, the PCMH model has been shown to reduce overall costs. Community Care of North Carolina, for example, leveraged a medical home approach to save $435 million for the state's Medicaid and SCHIP programs. Geisinger Health System (which includes a health plan) estimated its net savings from its PCMH model at $3.7 million, for a return on investment of more than two to one. And the Johns Hopkins PCMH program realized annual net Medicare savings of $1,364 per patient.[12]

Recently, the Patient-Centered Primary Care Collaborative (PCPCC), a stakeholder organization that advocates for the PCMH, released a summary of the peer-reviewed evidence in favor of this care delivery approach. According to the PCPCC:

- 61% of studies report cost reductions as a result of medical homes
- 61% report fewer emergency department visits
- 31% report fewer inpatient visits
- 13% report fewer readmissions
- 31% report improved access
- 23% report improved patient satisfaction
- 31% report an increase in preventive services
- 31% report improvements in population health[13]

Two key challenges

For medical homes to be successful in improving the quality and reducing the cost of care, they need the cooperation of outside specialists and hospitals. Yet the other providers in a PCMH's "medical neighborhood" may not be inclined to cooperate, because their incentives are not necessarily aligned with PCMH goals.[14] While the PCMH is designed to manage population health and avoid unnecessary care, the revenue of specialists and hospitals depends on the volume of services they provide. While these incentives are beginning to change with the evolution of value-based reimbursement, the transformation of the health-care payment system still has a long way to go.

Because of this barrier, some experts say, PCMHs cannot achieve their full potential unless they are incorporated into ACOs.[15] The latter organizations not only have the same incentives that medical homes do, but they are also comprised of both primary care physicians and specialists. So, whether multispecialty groups, independent practice associations, or health-care systems sponsor ACOs, they should, in theory, foster cooperation between the PCMH and its medical neighborhood.

Conversely, some observers view the PCMH as an essential building block of ACOs. That is because ACOs must be primary care-driven and patient-centered—the key characteristics of PCMHs—in order to succeed in a risk-bearing environment.[16]

Another key to the success of both PCMHs and ACOs is the automation of population health management. The goal of population health management is to keep patients as healthy as possible, thereby reducing the need for expensive ER visits, hospitalizations, and procedures.[17] As will be explained later, it is impossible for providers to manage population health effectively without the use of automation tools such as patient registries and analytic and care-management applications.

PCMH background

There are many definitions of the patient-centered medical home. One of the best comes from David Nash, MD, dean of the Jefferson School of Population Health at Jefferson University in Philadelphia:

> The patient-centered medical home (PCMH) is essentially delivery of holistic primary care based on ongoing, stable relationships between patients and their personal physicians. It is characterized by physician-directed integrated care teams, coordinated care, improved quality through the use of disease registries and health information technology, and enhanced access to care.[18]

A March 2007 joint statement by medical societies representing pediatricians, family physicians, and internists calls the PCMH "an approach to providing comprehensive primary care for children, youth and adults."[19] The chief components of the PCMH include

- a personal physician who is the first contact for his or her patients and who provides continuous and comprehensive care;
- a physician-led care team that takes collective responsibility for care;
- a "whole person" orientation, meaning that the personal physician will provide for all of a patient's health needs and arrange referrals to other health professionals as needed;

- care coordination across all care settings, facilitated by information technology and health information exchange;
- an emphasis on delivering high-quality, safe care in partnership with patients and their families;
- enhanced access to care through open scheduling, expanded hours, and improved communication among physicians, staff, and patients via secure e-mail and other modes; and
- additional reimbursement to reflect the value of the PCMH's activities and the costs of setting up the necessary infrastructure.

NCQA has further defined the PCMH by establishing a set of criteria that practices must meet to become NCQA-certified medical homes. These criteria have become increasingly important because most PCMH demonstration projects use them as a measurement tool,[20] and some health plans require NCQA certification for incentive payments to practices.[21]

Medical home certification

The medical home certification process grew out of another NCQA program that recognizes physicians for effectively using information technology and managing population health,[22] and the PCMH certification criteria also focus on health IT. The NCQA standards measure access and communication, patient tracking and registry functions, care management, patient self-management support, electronic prescribing, test tracking, referral tracking, performance reporting and improvement, and advanced electronic communications.[23]

Specifically, the NCQA's 2014 criteria for recognition as a PCMH consist of 26 elements in six domains, as follows:

1) Patient-Centered Access
    —Patient-centered appointment access
    —24/7 access to clinical advice
    —Electronic access

2) Team-Based Care
    —Continuity
    —Medical home responsibilities
    —Culturally and linguistically appropriate services
    —The practice team

3) Population Health Management
    —Patient information
    —Clinical data
    —Comprehensive health assessment
    —Use data for population health management
    —Implement evidence-based decision support

4) Care Management and Support
    —Identify patients for care management
    —Care planning and self-care support
    —Medication management
    —Use electronic prescribing
    —Support self-care and shared decision making

5) Care Coordination and Care Transitions
    —Test tracking and follow-up
    —Referral tracking and follow-up
    —Coordination care transitions

6) Performance Measurement and Quality Improvement
    —Measure clinical quality performance
    —Measure patient/family performance
    —Implement continuous quality improvement
    —Demonstrate continuous quality improvement
    —Report performance
    —Use certified EHR technology[24]

A quick glance at these criteria shows the importance of health IT in gaining recognition as a PCMH. In fact, several of the requirements, such as sending an electronic summary of care records to other providers in more than 50 percent of referrals, mirror the criteria for Meaningful Use stage 2. It's also notable that "must-pass" NCQA requirements such as "use data for population health management," "care planning and self-care support," and "referral tracking and follow-up" all necessitate the use of robust EHRs and ancillary applications.

In June 2012, NCQA announced plans to launch a specialty practice recognition program that will encourage specialists to work more closely with primary care practices to coordinate care—in other words, to make the medical neighborhood more friendly to medical homes. Again, health IT plays a prominent role in the criteria, many of which are aligned with the Meaningful Use stage 2 requirements.[25]

Challenges and solutions

To do population health management, a patient-centered medical home must build a number of core competencies. The care team in the practice must ensure that patients receive the preventive and chronic care recommended in evidence-based guidelines, that patients' conditions are tracked in a systematic way, that the practice reaches out to noncompliant patients and those who don't regularly see their doctor, that the practice provides patient education and self-management coaching, and that steps are taken to address poor health behaviors.

Because relatively few physician practices operate in this mode, the systematic application of population health management has been largely left to employers, health plans, and disease-management companies. The patient-centered medical home represents, in part, an effort to make physicians and patients central to this process. The Agency for Healthcare Research and Quality (AHRQ) has even coined a term for this new approach: practice-based population health (PBPH).[26]

A 2008 study of the preparedness of large group practices to become medical homes showed that most lacked key elements of the required infrastructure and practice approach.[27] Yet these groups have far more resources to make the necessary changes than small practices do. A recent study showed that small and medium-sized groups (under ten doctors) have only about one-fifth of the capabilities required in a PCMH.[28]

This is not to say that small practices cannot become medical homes. Some have achieved amazing feats of self-transformation. But even if they already have EHRs, small practices may not be able to afford other PCMH components, such as dedicated care coordinators and care managers. To expand their hours and provide after-hours access to patients, they must incur additional labor costs. And, as previously noted, they may find it difficult to persuade specialists and hospitals to cooperate with them on care coordination unless their incentives are aligned with the PCMH.

In the AAFP's TransforMED pilot, which ran from 2006 to 2008, the three dozen participating practices—some of them quite small—managed to achieve a number of PCMH goals. However, a report on their efforts pointed out that the pace of change is exhausting for practices and that they must have an "adaptive reserve" to keep going down the path of self-transformation. In addition, the report underlined the difficulty that doctors may have in assuming new roles vis-à-vis their staff.[29]

Experts have made several suggestions about how smaller practices might be able to turn themselves into medical homes.[30] One possibility is to use the kind of "practice transformation" consultants that were available to half of the practices in the TransforMED pilot. The government could also create regional extension centers, akin to or perhaps including the health IT RECs that have been used successfully in the Meaningful Use program, to help doctors over the hump. And both North Carolina and Vermont have successfully used community resource centers to supply shared care-coordination services that small practices could not afford on their own.[31]

Building the medical neighborhood

While these approaches might help practices build medical homes, their success as PCMHs will still be determined by how well they can build communication and collaboration channels with other providers. The potential role of ACOs in this area has already been mentioned. But it may not be necessary to wait until ACOs are widespread to begin improving the ecosystem in which the PCMH operates.

Under a $20.75-million grant from the Center for Medicare and Medicaid Innovation, VHA Inc., the national health-care network, TransforMED, and Phytel, a technology company that specializes in automated, provider-led population health-improvement solutions, are working together on a project to expand the PCMH concept to the patient-centered medical neighborhood. The goal is to connect acute-care hospitals with primary care, specialty, and subspecialty practices to deliver higher-quality, more patient-centered care at an affordable cost.[32]

VHA, TransforMED, and Phytel anticipate that their combined work across fifteen communities will save Medicare up to $53 million over a three-year period. TransforMED, the leading PCMH expert, will apply Phytel's population health-management solutions, and VHA will contribute its knowledge of quality management and ambulatory-care strategies for hospitals.

How much will it cost?

Most PCMH demonstrations sponsored by health plans use a mixed or hybrid payment model to reimburse physicians for the extra work and expense of providing a medical home. They pay physicians fee-for-service for the clinical work they do, plus a fixed care-coordination payment for each patient and some kind of quality incentive. While other approaches have been suggested, little data exist on how well they might work in encouraging PCMH activities.[33]

There's also no agreement on how high the care-coordination fee should be in the hybrid model. For example, the North Carolina Medicaid program paid primary-care doctors a coordination fee of $2.50 per patient per month.[34] In contrast, in a multi-payer pilot in Pennsylvania, the state required payments of $4 per patient per month to practices that had attained level 3 NCQA certification as medical homes.[35] Some estimates of appropriate care-coordination fees are much higher.[36]

One reason for the uncertainty about these fees is that not much is known about the costs of establishing a PCMH. A recent study of federally funded community health centers found that a fully functioning PCMH was associated with an operating cost per patient per month that was 4.6 percent higher than the cost of operating a similar center without a PCMH. The costs of tracking patients and improving quality—both health IT-intensive tasks—were particularly high. In total, the community health centers that functioned as medical homes added $2.26 per patient per month in operating costs, or about $500,000 per month for the average clinic.[37]

But the authors observed that another study of an integrated delivery system's use of a PCMH showed that it saved $18 per patient per month in averted hospitalizations and ER visits. Most of those savings accrued to payers, indicating a need for reimbursement sufficient to cover the infrastructure costs of PCMHs.

As noted earlier, some PCMHs that are part of integrated delivery systems have lowered costs and achieved a return on investment. But it's unclear whether that model would work for smaller, unaffiliated practices. What is clear is that the cost of creating and maintaining a medical home could be much lower if the practices were highly automated.

This approach requires the intelligent use of health information technology. By linking together some currently available health IT tools, physician groups can automate much of the work that might otherwise be too costly and difficult for them to do. Moreover, automating the manual processes of care coordination and care management makes it possible to scale the medical home to practices of every size.

Role of information technology

Observers agree that information technology, including the EHR, is essential to the patient-centered medical home's success. But EHRs lack some of the features required to do practice-based population health. AHRQ cites the inability of most EHRs to generate population-based reports easily, to present alerts and reminders in such a way that providers will use them rather than turning them off, to capture sufficiently detailed data on preventive care, and to interoperate with other clinical information systems.[38]

EHR vendors are moving to correct these deficiencies. For example, some applications allow users to adjust the level of alerts to their own needs and tolerance levels. And while another report points to the difficulty of using the registries imbedded in some EHRs,[39] those are also being improved to help physicians meet the Meaningful Use criteria.

Nevertheless, practices need a variety of health IT tools beyond EHRs to meet AHRQ's requirements for PBPH.[40] These requirements include the ability to

- identify subpopulations of patients,
- examine detailed characteristics of identified subpopulations,
- create reminders for patients and providers,
- track performance measures, and
- make data available in multiple forms.

Automation tools

A growing number of practices use external, web-based registries to supplement their EHRs. These registries compile lists of subpopulations that need particular kinds of preventive and chronic care, such as annual mammograms for women over 40 or HbA1c tests at particular intervals for diabetic patients. The continuously updated data in the registries comes from EHRs, practice management systems, labs, and pharmacies.

Evidence-based clinical protocols, which can be customized by physician practices, trigger alerts in the registries. When a registry is linked to an outbound messaging system, patients are notified by automated telephone, e-mail, or text messages to contact their physician for an appointment. Some registries can also send actionable data to care teams prior to patient visits.[41]

To be an effective tool for population health management, a registry should include all of a practice's patients. It should also have a sophisticated rules engine that combines disparate types of data with evidence-based guidelines, generating reports that provide many different views of the information. For example, the entire patient population could be filtered by payer, activity center, provider, health condition, and care gaps. The same filters could be applied to patients with a particular condition, such as diabetes, to find out where the practice needs to improve its diabetes care and to prepare actionable reports for care teams on individual patients.

Other IT tools that will also be important include online health risk assessments, automated education materials and health coaching, automation of actionable data for care teams, automation of care-management reports, and biometric home monitoring of patients with serious conditions. The accompanying table shows how information technology can be used to automate population health management.

Identification of Automation Opportunities in Manual Care-Management Process

Care-Team Process Step for "At-Risk" Patients	Manual Tasks	Automation Opportunities
1. Identify "at-risk" patients	• Review charts of patients scheduled for upcoming office visit • Review charts of patients associated with a specific payer contract with "pay-for-performance" incentives	• Utilize algorithms and data mining to identify all patients within provider panel with care gaps, irrespective of visit date or payer • Stratify and prioritize patients based on risk evaluation algorithms
2. Document gaps in care	• Review multiple screens and fields within EMR and Patient Management System to identify care gaps and appointment dates • Review paper charts for additional information	• Create reports across multiple sources of data for entire provider panel population to identify care gaps based on evidence-based algorithms • Flag patients with upcoming visits
3. Communicate gaps in care to treating providers	• Discuss gaps in care with provider as part of visit preparation process • Prepare cover sheet for paper chart	• Automate provider-level reports on patients with care gaps • Automate creation of patient care summaries for use in visit and between-visit management
4. Communicate treatment needs to patients	• Make phone calls to patients, often by nurses as well as other staff, which only reach a limited number of patients • Mail reminder letters for preventive care	• Utilize automated technologies to generate outreach by phone, e-mail, or text according to patient preference for all patients in provider panel with preventive or chronic-care gaps

Care-Team Process Step for "At-Risk" Patients	Manual Tasks	Automation Opportunities
5. Assessment of "at-risk" patients	• Conduct assessments during office visits or over the phone using paper or other tool that may or may not integrate with EMR	• Send all patients online health risk assessment tool; results can be used for individual and population management activities • Offer online health risk assessment part of patient portal
6. Educate patients about treatment plan and care needs	• Generate printout of patient treatment plan at end of visit; may be handed to patient or mailed • Make phone calls to patients for treatment plan follow-up	• Offer patient treatment plans and education tools through secure patient portal for ongoing patient support • Push reminders and other communications to individual and subpopulations of patients through patient portal as well as phone, e-mail, and text

Health risk assessment (HRA) is fundamental, because it serves as the basis for the interventions to be applied to patient populations. HRAs enable practices to sort their patients into four categories: healthy people, people at risk of or in early stages of chronic diseases, people with advanced chronic diseases, and those who are highly complex and at high risk for acute or adverse events. These groups are always changing. Those who are well today may be sick tomorrow, and those who have an early stage of disease today may be in a more advanced stage tomorrow. So regular administration of HRAs can help keep medical homes apprised of which patients are likely to need additional care in the future.

To reinforce the lifestyle modification messages delivered in the office visit, medical homes should use tailored communications and interventions to achieve and sustain behavior change. These include online educational materials that may be linked to HRAs, along with automated reminders to patients. Practices can also take advantage of the new mobile technologies, such as smartphones and texting, as well as patient web portals that may be attached to EHRs.

Medical homes can also use automation tools to support the efficient functioning of care teams. These include accurate and usable patient data summaries to minimize the need for chart reviews. The summaries, generated by registries, will remind providers of a patient's care gaps and the need to work with him or her on modifying health behavior. Care teams can also streamline the visit preparation process by identifying care opportunities and having patients get tests done before visits.

To support the work flow of care managers, medical homes can deploy software that automatically sets priorities for their communications with patients, based on the severity of their condition. Using data from EHRs and registries, this type of application can tell a care manager whether he or she needs to call a patient directly or whether electronic messaging will suffice.

Biometric home monitoring, which has been around for more than a decade, is finally starting to get some financial support from health plans.[42] As a result, it may be feasible for medical homes to start using it to keep tabs on their sickest patients with such chronic conditions as heart failure, diabetes, and high-risk pregnancy. Because doctors don't have time to monitor the continuous stream of data, this would be a natural task for care coordinators.

The benefits of using these health IT tools include the ability to track, monitor, and engage patients; to tailor interventions to different segments of the population; to measure performance for quality reporting; to automate care coordination; to ensure that care gaps are filled; and to do all of this without increasing the workload of doctors or staff members.

Conclusion

The patient-centered medical home is a work in progress. Much remains to be learned about the most effective techniques for building and maintaining a PCMH. But three conclusions can already be drawn from the pilots that have already been done: successful medical homes will have to perform population health management; they will need a variety of health IT tools to do that and to coordinate care effectively; and they will have to develop relationships and work flows with the other providers in their medical neighborhoods.

Major changes in practice work flow and work roles must accompany the proper use of information technology. In the end, practices must be completely reengineered to provide effective, patient-centered medical homes—and the environment in which they operate must also change to permit seamless care coordination. All of this change can be less painful and lead to more productive results if practices use the right combination of technologies to do population health management.

The NCQA's decision to base many of its criteria on the Meaningful Use Stage 2 requirements is indicative of the close connection between practice transformation and Meaningful Use. In the next chapter, we show where the government's Meaningful Use program is driving the health-care system and how that will affect providers' PHM strategies.

Section 2

How to Get There

Chapter 4

Meaningful Use and Population Health Management

- *Introduction*: The government's EHR incentive program is designed to transform health-care delivery and dovetails with other health-care reform initiatives. Population health management, the goal of these initiatives, requires advanced forms of health IT.
- *Meaningful Use overview*: From the beginning, the requirements for showing Meaningful Use of EHRs have emphasized population health management. A brief description of the Meaningful Use program is offered.
- *PHM components of MU*: The MU stage 2 criteria and proposed stage 3 criteria have numerous components related to PHM. These are summarized here, along with observations about how automation tools can help providers show MU and manage population health.
- *Health information exchange*: The stage 2 and 3 requirements emphasize the need for providers to exchange patient data with one another. Many physicians and hospitals are finding this challenging, because the mechanisms for information exchange are still being developed in many areas.
- *Patient-generated data:* Some menu items in the proposed stage 3 criteria relate to patient-generated data, including health risk assessments and functional status reports. These are controversial but essential to patient engagement and risk management. Some

observers note that telemonitoring and mHealth data should also be considered as patient-generated data.

The government's EHR incentive program, which has disbursed nearly $23 billion so far, has greatly increased the adoption and use of EHRs by doctors and hospitals in the last four years.[1] Because of the criteria used to reward providers for the "meaningful use" of EHRs, the initiative has also promoted the use of that technology to transform health-care delivery.

The Meaningful Use program, as it has come to be known, did not evolve in isolation from other aspects of health-care reform. The Patient Protection and Affordable Care Act of 2010 (ACA), for example, includes a number of provisions that presuppose the widespread adoption of EHRs and some degree of interoperability among disparate systems.

Among these are the provisions that set up the Medicare Shared Savings Program (MSSP) for accountable care organizations and the CMS Innovation Center, which is charged with testing, evaluating, and expanding new care-delivery models.[2] Among the innovation center's initiatives are a bundled-payment demonstration and CMS's Comprehensive Primary Care Initiative. In addition, CMS is involved in multiple pilots of the patient-centered medical home.[3] All of these initiatives are oriented to population health management and require the use of advanced health IT.

Meaningful Use overview

The HITECH provisions of the 2009 American Recovery and Reinvestment Act (ARRA), which established the Meaningful Use program, have these objectives:

- Improve quality, safety, and efficiency and reduce health disparities.
- Engage patients and their families in their health care.
- Improve care coordination.

- Ensure privacy and confidentiality for personal health information.
- Improve population health.[4]

The HITECH legislation did not describe how these aims were to be achieved. But it did direct the Department of Health and Human Services (HHS) to include electronic prescribing, health information, and quality data reporting among the requirements for receiving EHR incentives.[5]

The initial MU regulations, published in July 2010, included a framework for moving toward population health management (PHM), although some of the PHM-related requirements were made optional or were postponed to stages 2 or 3 of Meaningful Use. Examples of PHM-related criteria in stage 1 include showing the ability to exchange data with other providers, generating lists of patients with specific conditions to use in quality-improvement activities, and sending reminders to patients for preventive or follow-up care.[6]

Overall, the stage 1 criteria focus on electronically capturing health information in a coded format, using that data to track key clinical conditions, communicating that information for purposes of care coordination, implementing clinical-decision support tools, and reporting clinical quality measures and public health information.

In stage 2, the requirements for EPs and hospitals have been expanded "to encourage the use of health IT for continuous quality improvement at the point of care and the exchange of information in the most structured format possible, such as the electronic transmission of orders entered using computerized provider order entry (CPOE) and the electronic transmission of diagnostic test results."

The stage 3 criteria are expected to "focus on promoting improvements in quality, safety and efficiency, focusing on decision support for national high priority conditions, patient access to self management tools, access to comprehensive patient data, and improving population health."[7]

Meaningful Use 101

The basics of the Meaningful Use program are fairly well-known at this point. But we will briefly summarize its essential provisions to clarify the discussion for those who are unfamiliar with the program.

Both eligible hospitals and eligible professionals—who include physicians and some other types of health-care professionals—must show Meaningful Use of certified EHR technology to receive incentive payments and avoid penalties later on. There are two MU programs, one through Medicare and the other through Medicaid. Providers who participate in the Medicare MU program are eligible to receive nearly $44,000 in total incentive payments, while nearly $64,000 is available to providers who qualify for and show Meaningful Use in the Medicaid program. Providers cannot receive payments from both programs at the same time.[8]

The time lines for the two programs are different. Under Medicare, EPs have been allowed to attest to stage 1 of Meaningful Use since April 2011. They attest each year to receive incremental payments for up to five years and avoid later penalties in the form of lower Medicare payments. The last year in which providers can attest to Meaningful Use for the first time is 2014.[9]

Medicaid providers can receive a first-year payment if they adopt, implement, or upgrade EHRs without showing Meaningful Use. They must begin to demonstrate Meaningful Use by 2016.[10]

In the Medicare program, Meaningful Use stage 2 began in January 2014 and extends through 2016. Stage 3 will begin in 2017.[11] The penalty phase for those who did not attest to MU by 2013 and do not qualify for a hardship exception starts in 2015, and the reductions in Medicare reimbursement grow in subsequent years.[12] However, a rule change proposed in May 2014, following a lackluster start to stage 2, would allow providers who are having difficulty in obtaining new certified EHRs or attesting to stage 2 objectives to attest to stage 1 criteria in 2014.[13]

The requirements for Meaningful Use are divided into core objectives that providers must satisfy and an optional menu from which they must select a certain number of objectives. In MU stage 1, for example, EPs had fifteen core objectives and had to select five of ten menu items.[14]

Certification bodies approved by the Office of the National Coordinator for Health IT (ONC) can certify both complete EHRs and modular components of EHRs as meeting ONC's criteria.[15] This regulation allows the certification of various nontraditional EHRs and supplemental technologies that can aid physicians in improving quality and obtaining government incentives.

The certification requirements adopted in 2011 reflected the MU stage 1 criteria. Under CMS's current regulations, starting in 2014, providers who attest to MU stage 1 or 2 must have EHRs that meet ONC's 2014-edition requirements. The new proposed rule would allow providers to use certified EHR technology that meets 2011 or 2014 requirements or a combination of the two, but only in 2014.[16]

Upping the ante in stages 2 and 3

The MU stage 2 requirements are considerably stiffer than those of stage 1. While the total numbers of core and menu objectives are similar to those in stage 1—twenty for EPs and nineteen for EHs—some of these goals and the associated measures are far more difficult to meet.[17]

All but one of the menu objectives in stage 1 are required items in stage 2. Also, data fields that had to be completed in stage 1, such as problem and medication lists, have been merged into a summary record of care that includes many other data elements. EPs have two new core objectives related to patient engagement, including secure messaging with patients and ensuring that 5 percent of patients view, download, or transmit health records that are available online. There are also new health information exchange criteria that are discussed below.[18]

Besides these challenges and new quality measures, many providers must also cope with their vendors' delays in making available 2014-certified EHRs that they can use to attest to Meaningful Use. CMS has created a new hardship exception to help providers caught in this bind from being penalized. But the meaning of this exception is still unclear, and some providers are being forced to switch EHRs because their vendors have not gotten their EHRs certified under the 2014 edition.[19]

Meanwhile, the Health IT Policy Committee (HITPC), which advises ONC on Meaningful Use, recently approved a draft proposal on the stage 3 criteria. After reviewing the recommendations, ONC and CMS are expected to release a proposed rule on stage 3 in fall 2014.[20]

The HITPC proposal suggests adoption of several new menu measures, including a measure on providing electronic notifications of significant health-care events to a patient's care team and a measure requiring hospitals and health systems to accept patient-generated data. The four main areas of emphasis in stage 3, according to the proposal, will be clinical-decision support, patient engagement, care coordination, and population health.[21]

PHM components of Meaningful Use

EHRs were not originally designed for population health management. They were supposed to help physicians document better, reduce recordkeeping costs, and justify higher evaluation and management charges. While EHRs always had some safety and quality features, such as drug-interaction checkers and health-maintenance alerts, these were very limited. Moreover, the lack of interoperability among disparate EHRs has made it difficult for providers to exchange information with each other.

The 2014 certification rules have forced vendors to augment their systems in certain ways, and some leading EHR companies have added population health-management features. But ancillary applications can still make a big difference in the ability of providers to show Meaningful Use and improve the quality of care.

What follows are some Meaningful Use stage 2 requirements and stage 3 proposals that could help EPs manage population health.[22,23] In addition, we note where supplemental applications might help EPs meet the MU criteria. Bear in mind that only certified EHR technology can be used to show Meaningful Use. Some care-management tools, such as automated patient messaging applications, have been certified. But even if a supplemental application can't be used for Meaningful Use, it could help health-care organizations improve population health.

Clinical-decision support

MU stage 2 requires EPs to use five clinical-decision support (CDS) rules, other than drug-interaction alerts; the stage 3 proposal mandates the use of CDS rules in at least four of six National Quality Strategy areas, including drug-interaction checking. Health-maintenance alerts in EHRs can meet the criteria for CDS alerts to improve preventive and chronic care, but they fall short of what's needed for PHM.

For example, these alerts often can't be customized; in some applications, users must build them from scratch; and they're usually not linked to automated messaging or PHM dashboards. Use of an outside registry and protocol-linked software would give providers the tools they need both for PHM and to help them meet the CDS requirement of Meaningful Use.

Patient access to records

In stage 2, more than 50 percent of patients seen during the reporting period must be able to view, download, and transmit their health information online within four days after it becomes available to the EP. Five percent of patients must actually do so.

In the stage 3 proposal, EPs and EHs must give patients the ability to view/download/transmit their health information within twenty-four hours after a visit, and test results must be provided online within four days.

The care summary requirement in stage 3 remains the same as in stage 2, except that instructions pertaining to the visit must also be included.

Patient-generated information

In a proposed stage 3 menu item, EPs and EHs would have to receive provider-requested, patient-generated health information through either secure messaging or a structured or semi-structured questionnaire. The latter could include screening questionnaires, medication-adherence surveys, intake forms, health risk assessments (HRAs), or functional-status surveys.

Patient-generated health data would represent a big leap forward for population health management. Not only would it be easier to track the health status of patients who have not recently visited their provider, but the inclusion of HRAs could also help organizations measure the health risks of individuals.

Patient-specific education

In stage 2, EPs and EHs must use their EHRs to identify patient-specific education resources and provide those resources to patients. In stage 3, they must also provide the educational materials in a non-English-speaking patient's preferred language, where they are available.

The selection and provision of these resources should be automated to save time and effort. The EHR can use clinical protocols to identify the correct materials, and patients can be sent secure messages with links to the websites where those resources can be found. Where the EHR doesn't have this end-to-end capability, outside applications may be utilized.

Secure messaging

In stage 2, EPs must use secure electronic messaging to communicate with at least 5 percent of patients seen during the reporting period. That remains the same in the stage 3 proposal, and certified EHRs must also be able to track responses to patient-generated messages. This objective is important in PHM because it provides a key vehicle for follow-up care between visits.

Patient reminders

In stages 2 and 3, more than 10 percent of patients who have had two or more office visits to an EP within the previous twenty-four months must receive reminders for preventive and follow-up care. The EHR must be used to identify the patients who should receive reminders, which can be provided online or printed out, depending on patient preference.

Many patients want to receive these reminders online, but EHRs are not set up to send messages automatically. This is where an automated patient-outreach service could be used to reach patients by secure e-mail, secure texting, or phone.

Condition-specific lists

Stages 1 and 2 both require the ability to generate lists of patients by specific conditions to use for quality improvement, reduction of disparities, research, or outreach. Certified EHRs can do this, but this functionality is severely limited for purposes of PHM. A robust outside registry can produce far more specific subgroup lists for use in care management and disease management.

Transitions of care

When a patient is discharged from a hospital or emergency department or referred to a specialist, the EP or EH that transitions or refers the patient to another provider is required to provide a summary of care in both stages 2 and 3. This summary record must be provided in any form for more than 50 percent of patients, and electronically for 10 percent of patients. In the stage 3 proposal, the types of transitions are described in more detail, and organizations are encouraged to include narrative notes, patient goals, and patient instructions.

Along with medication reconciliation at transitions of care, the summary record requirement helps ensure smooth handoffs that are essential for good care coordination and for the ability of medical homes to function well within their medical neighborhoods.

Notification of significant events

A new proposed menu requirement in stage 3 requires eligible hospitals to send electronic notifications of significant health events within four hours to members of the patient's care team. These events include arrival at an ED, admission to a hospital, discharge from an ED or hospital, and death. For organizations that seek to coordinate care and manage population health, these notifications are essential.

Other requirements

The stage 2 requirements and the stage 3 proposal also place a strong emphasis on transmitting vaccination data to immunization registries and reporting syndromic surveillance and reportable lab data to public health agencies. HITPC considers these requirements to be integral to population health management.

Health information exchange

A key goal of MU stage 2—as well as of the new care-delivery models—is to improve the exchange of patient information between providers who have disparate EHR systems. Besides having to exchange care summaries at transitions of care, providers must also do this at least once with an EHR that is different from their own. The stage 3 proposal doesn't go beyond this, but an overarching goal enunciated in the CMS blueprint for stage 3 is to provide "access to comprehensive patient data." HITPC might not have pursued that explicitly because the technology isn't mature enough yet, but it still remains the ultimate objective.

Many health-care providers are having difficulty in meeting even the fairly limited requirement for health information exchange in MU stage 2. One reason is that the mechanisms for information exchange are still being developed in many areas. Despite having received more than half a billion dollars in federal aid, statewide health information organizations (HIOs) and the regional exchanges that some of them support have not gained much traction outside of a few states, such as Delaware, Indiana, Michigan, and New York. In contrast, private HIOs created by health-care organizations have grown dramatically in recent years.[24]

Nevertheless, a recent survey reveals that more than six in ten hospitals are now exchanging data with providers outside of their enterprises—a 51 percent increase since 2008. While many of those hospitals are just exchanging lab and radiology reports with outside providers (57 percent and 58 percent, respectively), 42 percent exchange clinical-care summaries and 37 percent exchange medication histories.[25]

Whether health-care organizations are doing this because it saves money or because of Meaningful Use stage 2 is beside the point. What's important is that increased electronic connectivity will help them manage population health.

Health information organizations are also essential to PHM, because they allow care teams to look up information on their patients in other providers' systems and, conversely, to obtain data on patients they've never seen before. The latter ability is especially important in emergency departments, which treat many patients who have not been seen by anyone else in their organizations. In addition, providers can use HIOs to find out what other providers have done for their patients.[26]

Providers can also exchange health information by using the Direct secure-messaging protocol, which allows them to send messages and attached documents directly to one another. Direct is becoming more popular as the health information service providers (HISPs) that convey the messages get accredited and start to form a national network.[27] But Direct only allows data to be "pushed" from one point to another. HIOs are necessary for data to be "pulled" out of multiple databases.

HIOs can support or enhance many of the functions required in MU stage 2, notes a report from the Health Information Management and Systems Society (HIMSS). Most significant from the viewpoint of MU is the ability of HIOs to exchange care summaries at transitions of care.[28]

Patient-generated data

The inclusion of patient-generated data in MU stage 3 is controversial—which is one reason why the draft proposal makes it a menu item. Many health-care providers are not used to considering patient-generated data beyond the items that patients fill out on a clipboard during the intake process. By and large, physicians are not amenable to the idea of having patients correct or update their health information. And there are still many questions about how best to integrate patient-entered data in the EHR.

Yet increasing the participation of patients in their own health care is a key element of Meaningful Use and of population health management. Without patient engagement, it's doubtful that population health can be significantly improved.

Some organizations, such as Group Health Cooperative of Puget Sound, are having patients fill out health risk assessments, and Dartmouth Hitchcock Spine Clinic collects health status information from patients before each visit. But this is far from a mainstream approach.[29]

An ONC report on patient-generated health data notes that it can be very important for the new care-delivery systems, including ACOs and patient-centered medical homes. These new delivery models depend on patient engagement and on care teams working with patients between office visits, the report notes. "It therefore becomes more critical to value the patient as a source of vital information."[30]

The American Health Information Management Association (AHIMA) has also weighed in on the inclusion of patient-generated health data in the MU stage 3 proposal. Besides the use of patient-entered data, an AHIMA blog post points out, "One growing source of patient-generated data is from an expanding array of eHealth tools that patients and their families are adopting to aid them in the management of their health." These include both remote patient monitoring and mobile health applications, AHIMA notes.[31]

Conclusion

Meaningful Use is at a crossroads, with some observers expressing doubt that a substantial percentage of providers will continue on to stages 2 and 3.[32,33] Yet to the extent that doctors and hospitals persevere and EHR vendors provide them with the means to do so, Meaningful Use has the potential to create much of the infrastructure needed for population health management.

Even if they eschew Meaningful Use in the future, health-care organizations must build this infrastructure to prepare for value-based reimbursement, which requires them to manage population health. Either way, the basic ingredients of PHM—patient engagement, care coordination, health information exchange, and automated care management—will require sophisticated health IT tools that go beyond the EHR as we know it today.

These tools are also essential to wiring together providers in clinically integrated networks (CINs). These CINs enable providers in disparate practices and health systems to work together as care teams that can coordinate care and ensure the whole patient population is managed efficiently. Chapter 5 explains how.

Integrating Data across a Clinically Integrated Network

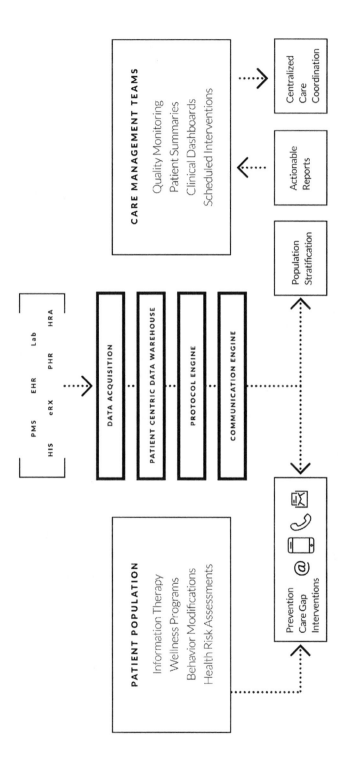

Chapter 5

Clinically Integrated Networks

- *Introduction*: Clinical integration of providers must come before ACOs and population health management. But most organizations lack the key components of clinical integration, including a robust IT infrastructure.
- *Clinically integrated networks*: The FTC and Justice Department allow these networks to negotiate with payers if they're designed to raise quality and lower costs. This is important to health-care organizations that want to build ACOs that include outside physician groups. If they form a CIN first, it must be able to integrate data from multiple EHRs to manage cost and quality.
- *Automation tools*: To manage population health successfully, CINs must deploy automation tools that allow them to use their care managers effectively. They must also have solutions that enable them to engage all of their patients and follow up on those that have been recently discharged from the hospital. Finally, they must be able to measure the performance of their providers.
- *Conclusion*: A successful CIN like Advocate Healthcare in Chicago took many years to develop. Health-care organizations that are preparing for value-based reimbursement don't have that much time. They should take advantage of the latest health IT solutions to accelerate the process.

More and more health-care organizations are recognizing that clinical integration of providers is a prerequisite to care coordination, population health management, and accountable care organizations. They also know that patient centered medical homes—the building blocks of ACOs—can thrive only in patient-centered medical neighborhoods where specialists collaborate with primary care physicians. For this cooperation to be truly effective, all of these providers must be clinically integrated.

The Premier Healthcare Alliance recently published a study of the capabilities of organizations in its ACO collaborative. According to the study, most of these health-care providers lacked the clinical integration they needed for ACO success.

> Given that clinical integration is the ability to coordinate appropriate care for the population served, this capability represented a significant gap across all organizations. Those organizations that did score higher definitely exhibited a greater ability to foster coordination and collaboration across the multiple healthcare providers during the patient's episode of care. Disease management programs are one example of such care coordination.[1]

The backbone of clinical integration is a robust health IT infrastructure. To enable care teams to deliver efficient, high-quality care, this infrastructure must consist of far more than networked electronic health records. Provider organizations must also deploy analytics and automation tools that make the data actionable in clinical work flows and that facilitate population health management. When properly integrated with EHRs and financial systems, these applications can enable organizations to scale up quickly for care management at a population-wide level and can provide them with the insights they need to take financial risk.

This chapter explains the components of clinical integration and summarizes the kinds of information technology required for its implementation. Case studies of organizations that are building the necessary infrastructure are also included.

Clinically integrated networks

Until recently, except in group-model HMOs such as Kaiser Permanente and Group Health Cooperative, and big multispecialty groups like the Mayo Clinic and the Cleveland Clinic, clinical integration was viewed primarily as a legal concept that allowed unrelated fee-for-service providers to negotiate joint contracts with payers. These providers often came together through vehicles such as physician-hospital organizations (PHOs) and independent practice associations (IPAs).

The Federal Trade Commission (FTC) and the Department of Justice initially regarded efforts by providers to negotiate together as per se violations of antitrust law that would lead to price fixing. But about twelve years ago, the agencies began to issue statements and rulings that carved out a legal space for clinically integrated networks to bargain with payers if their stated purpose was to improve quality and reduce costs. These opinions have continued to grow in scope over the years.[2]

In February 2013, for example, the FTC issued an advisory opinion permitting the operations of the Norman (Oklahoma) Physician Hospital Organization, a partnership between the Norman Regional Health System and the Norman Physicians Association. Although this clinically integrated network (CIN) planned to negotiate prices with payers, the FTC said that was unlikely to lead to a restraint of trade since the independent physicians were free to contract with health plans on their own.[3]

The FTC and the Department of Justice define a permissible CIN as "an active, ongoing program to evaluate and modify the clinical practice patterns of physician participants to create a high degree of interdependence and collaboration among the physicians to control costs and ensure quality."[4] Among the criteria for such a program, the agencies state, are the selection of high-quality providers, ownership and commitment by providers, physician investment in the program, appropriate use of health IT, collaboration in the care of patients, quality and cost-improvement initiatives, data collection and dissemination, and accountability.

As health-care organizations prepare for accountable care, these requirements have taken on a new importance. That is because few organizations encompass all of the providers they need to deliver comprehensive, integrated care to a population across all care settings. Even if health-care systems employ physicians, they usually need help from private-practice doctors and other unrelated providers in the community. That means that their clinically integrated networks must cross business boundaries and that unrelated providers will be bargaining with health plans on shared-savings and bundled-payment arrangements. To do that legally, they must abide by the federal rules.

Current definition

A CIN is a jointly governed group of providers, including independent physicians, physician groups, employed physicians, and hospitals or health systems, that work together to

- develop mechanisms to monitor and improve the utilization, cost, and quality of health-care services provided;
- develop and implement protocols and best practices;
- furnish higher-quality, more efficient care than could be achieved by working independently;
- pool infrastructure and human and financial resources; and
- jointly contract with commercial and government payers and employers on a shared-savings or financial-risk basis.[5]

This approach is especially important to health-care systems because their employed physician groups often do not include enough primary care physicians (PCPs) for a successful ACO. The CIN approach allows them to integrate outside PCPs with their employed doctors to create the proper balance of specialties. For example, Orlando Health in Orlando, Florida, employs 500 physicians, the bulk of them non-primary care specialists. To align community PCPs with its goals, Orlando Health has created a 400-doctor CIN that includes both employed and independent physicians and has partnered with the largest primary care group in central Florida.

According to the Premier ACO collaborative study, having more employed physicians was not associated with a more successful ACO strategy. "In fact, some of the highest performers had the lowest proportion of employed physicians."[6] So a clinical integration approach can be the best way to gear up for accountable care or value-based reimbursement.

Basic requirements

Successful clinical integration requires a tightly aligned, physician-governed network that uses a single set of performance metrics. Engaging physicians and getting them to agree on clinical protocols is not easy, but it is essential to clinical integration and a common approach to care management. The organization must also agree on how to measure utilization of resources and network financial performance.

The health IT infrastructure has to support not only performance measurement and reporting, but also the operational requirements of improving performance on cost, quality, and patient experience. To achieve these goals, it must be able to:

- interface multiple EHRs to a population health management platform, either directly or through a health information exchange;
- integrate lab, pharmacy, imaging, and other ancillary data;
- apply business and clinical intelligence to data in near-real time;
- provide a single view of patient data to providers and care managers;
- enable managers to pull up data quickly on subpopulations of patients; and
- generate performance assessments of individual providers, sites, specialties, and the entire organization.

Health-care organizations have some problems with claims data, which are out-of-date and often flawed. But at least for now, it is difficult for most organizations to get an accurate idea of how much care delivery costs them without some claims data from payers. In addition, this data can be useful in tracking out-of-network referrals.

Automation tools

Today's clinical integration networks must be able to do population health management to demonstrate their value to payers. CINs may use nurse care managers to perform tasks that require human intervention, such as working with high-risk patients and calling discharged patients who don't understand their discharge instructions. But to manage population health effectively, CINs need a high degree of automation, which allows them to provide appropriate care to every patient. Organizations cannot hire enough care managers to track, monitor, contact, and intervene with every patient who needs help if they rely on manual methods.[7]

The first step in creating a CIN health IT infrastructure is to aggregate data in a data warehouse. That is no different than what any health-care enterprise or group practice must do to get value from the data. But unlike an integrated group, a CIN consists of many different business entities that use disparate EHRs. So the CIN must have a strategy and the appropriate tools for mapping the data from many different sources to a single, normative database or a single view of data.

This mapping process must overcome numerous obstacles. For example, patients must be uniquely matched to the available data on them, and they must also be attributed correctly to their primary providers. This attribution is not easy when patients have multiple providers or frequently move from one physician to another. Also, the data has to be made actionable for patient engagement. That requires cleaning up the demographic data and contact information.

CINs must also verify and ensure the integrity of the clinical data, using special analytic tools. Part of the data aggregation and normalization process involves the identification of gaps and errors in the information. If the informaticians who do this see that certain data elements are missing or clearly out of range, they have to go back to the practice or the hospital that generated that data and find out why.

The health IT staffers in most health-care organizations are neither trained for nor have time to do this kind of work. Yet it is essential to clinical integration and population health management. So CINs may have to retain outside specialists who have the expertise and the right tools to complete this key step successfully.

Risk stratification

To automate population health management, support providers at the point of care, and increase the effectiveness of care management, CINs must apply analytics to the clinical data in their repositories and registries. This starts with risk stratification of patients into high-, medium-, and low-risk categories. Risk stratification can be used to assign patients to different kinds of interventions; in combination with predictive modeling software, it can also forecast which patients are most likely to get sick.[8]

Patient outreach

By applying clinical protocols to a registry, analytic tools can identify patients' preventive and chronic care needs. CINs can connect that solution with automated outbound messaging to remind patients when it is time for them to make appointments with their providers for necessary care. Such an approach has been shown to increase the likelihood that patients will seek the care they need.[9] It also provides value by reconnecting patients with their physicians after a long hiatus.

The same approach can be used as the basis of campaigns to get patients more engaged in their own care so that they will not have to see a provider. For example, automated messages could suggest that patients take specific steps to stop smoking or lose weight. This kind of outreach could be coordinated with public health campaigns directed at the same behavior change.

In terms of population health management, automated outreach is critical for preventing people from getting sick or sicker. All patients of the CIN's providers must be monitored and encouraged to seek appropriate care or take better care of themselves to optimize population health.

Care management

The automation of care management offers several advantages. First, outreach to keep low-risk patients on track can be done with a minimum of effort. Also, care managers can use automated care-gap identification to draw up work lists of high-risk individuals who need their attention. As for those at medium risk—chiefly people who have chronic diseases— care managers can use automation tools not only for outreach, but also for targeted interventions, such as educational campaigns, disease management, and arranging group visits.

In a mature CIN that has used these tools for some time, care managers can initiate hundreds of such campaigns by using the software to set parameters for people with different conditions and for subcategories of those populations. This approach can multiply the effectiveness of a single care manager manyfold. Early-stage CINs may want to start with priority conditions and expand from there to make sure their care teams are prepared for the influx of patients. The worst thing organizations can do is to tell patients they need care and then not be able to provide it to them in a reasonable time frame.

A CIN must create a unified care-management structure on behalf of all its member practices. While patients will view the care managers as an extension of their providers' practices, those nurses will actually perform care-management and patient-engagement tasks for the entire network. Similarly, the data that form the basis of the care managers' work lists will come from a central database, and the care managers will all use the same analytic and automation tools.

Patient engagement

This middle layer of technology between individual practices and the CIN can also be used to increase patient engagement. We have already mentioned automated patient outreach and educational campaigns. But that is only the beginning of the modalities that technology can facilitate. Among the other tools CINs can use to get patients more involved in their own health are online health risk assessments, mobile health apps, secure texting, and patient portals.

Patient portals can be used for record sharing, results delivery, appointment and refill requests, and online communication with providers. The use of these websites is soaring because providers need them to meet requirements of Meaningful Use stage 2 by sharing health records with their patients.[10] Portals attached to EHRs in physician practices can pose a problem, because patients would prefer not to download multiple records from different providers. So some CINs are beginning to create unified portals that offer a single point of contact to patients.

Nevertheless, CINs should not base their patient-engagement strategies on portals. Many providers do not yet have them, and many patients don't use them. Even at Kaiser Permanente, which has had a portal since 2005, only about 60 percent of members with website access use it regularly.[11] So automated messaging to patients—by phone, text, or e-mail—will continue to be an essential method of contacting patients who have care gaps or who need to be further engaged in their own care.

Post-discharge care

CINs must also have a way to follow up with patients after discharge from a hospital or an ED. One efficient way of doing that is to use automated messaging to survey patients within the first twenty-four hours after discharge to home. Using feedback from the survey calls, care managers can contact patients who have questions about their discharge instructions or their medications or who have not made an appointment with a primary care provider.

If hospitals wish, they can use the same mechanism to notify providers that their patients have been discharged and are in need of follow-up care. If a patient is having difficulty scheduling a doctor appointment, a care manager can contact his or her physician's practice and find out what the problem is.

Performance evaluation

Just like any health-care system or group practice, a CIN must be able to measure performance in order to improve it. This requires analytic tools that can evaluate performance at the level of individual providers and offices, as well as for the entire organization. Among the parameters that must be measured are quality, cost, utilization, and patient experience. In addition, CINs must be able to analyze adherence to protocols in the care of subpopulations, such as patients with type 2 diabetes or patients who have both type 2 diabetes and hypertension.

Before a CIN can measure performance, the providers in the network must agree on a set of clinical protocols that they are going to follow. This is a difficult but not insuperable challenge. As one study of clinical integration points out:

> For a new CI program, it can be difficult enough just to get physician buy-in for performance measurement, let alone for care pathways. But as CI programs develop stronger physician engagement, clinical standardization seems to become easier. Indeed, the challenge becomes less about winning physician buy-in and more about how the program can accelerate the standardization process across hundreds of conditions or diagnoses, many of which cut across specialty areas and care settings.[12]

Once a CIN has its protocols and its physicians have committed to following them, it can begin to measure how closely they adhere to those guidelines. CIN managers can also use dashboards based on clinical analytics to see how well their approaches to caring for certain subpopulations are working. If the percentage of diabetic patients with HbA1c > 9 does not fall over time, for instance, the medical director of a CIN can drill down into the data to find out why and do something about it. That might include talking to doctors who are outliers or creating automated campaigns to increase the engagement of patients who have diabetes.

Physicians must be able to view data on their own patient panels so they can see how well various segments of that population are doing and assess their own performance. A dashboard designed for providers should also give them access to data on individual patients so they can see which ones have care gaps or need interventions to improve their health.

Conclusion

Clinically integrated networks are still fairly new, although a few IPAs and PHOs have had success with this strategy for years. Among them is Advocate Physician Partners (APP), a cluster of PHOs associated with Advocate Healthcare in Chicago. APP has long held risk contracts from local payers, and its ACO has cut costs for Illinois Blue Cross and Blue Shield. The organization has also improved quality, safety, and patient satisfaction.[13]

Founded in 1995, APP took nearly a decade to fully develop its CIN. Lee Sacks, MD, chief medical officer of Advocate, told the *New York Times* recently, "It's hard to imagine you could start from scratch and do this and be successful in three years."[14]

Unfortunately, health-care organizations gearing up for accountable care today must move faster. So they will have to figure out new ways to do it. Part of the solution is for every provider in the CIN to use electronic health records—something that APP emphasized early on. But in addition, they need automation and analytic tools that can enable the CIN to scale up quickly for population health management.

Ultimately, the ability of providers to integrate clinically depends on effective physician governance and culture change. Financial incentives must be aligned, and doctors must be willing to give up some of their autonomy to work with other care providers as a team.

A robust health IT infrastructure is also a prerequisite for clinical integration. Solutions now exist to automate most of the routine tasks involved in population health management. CINs that use these tools can accelerate the process of becoming more tightly integrated and providing value in the marketplace.

CINs, ACOs, and other organizations capable of taking financial risk all need the ability to predict which patients are likely to get sick and the financial implications for the organization. To do this, providers are increasingly using the same kind of predictive modeling that health plans have long utilized. The next chapter describes these analytics and explains what they're being used for.

Case Study: Orlando Health

Orlando Health is a large health-care system that includes seven hospitals with a total of 1,800 beds. It employs 500 physicians, most of them specialists. To achieve its goal of becoming the highest-quality, lowest-cost provider in central Florida, Orlando Health needs to get additional primary care physicians on the team. So it has formed a clinically integrated network that includes its employed doctors, independent primary care physicians, and practitioners employed by the University of Florida health-care system. It has also become aligned with the largest primary care group in the region.

Meanwhile, Orlando Health is moving forward on several related fronts. It is participating in a CMS Medical Neighborhood demonstration project with VHA, TransforMED, and Phytel. Most of its ambulatory care offices are on their way to being recognized as patient-centered medical homes. And it has formed an ACO that has shared-savings contracts with CMS and private payers.

Early on, Orlando Health recognized that its clinical integration strategy required the use of automation tools for care management and patient engagement. After doing on-site demos and site visits with ten population health management vendors, it chose a company that offered an easy-to-use provider interface, snapshots of patient care gaps, the ability to interface with multiple EHRs, the ability to integrate pharmacy and lab data, and integrated patient outreach and education capabilities.

To do population health management across the continuum of care, Orlando Health's CIN also needs to build a health information exchange, and its physicians must agree on the clinical protocols that they're willing to follow and be evaluated on. In addition, its health IT infrastructure must be capable of reporting on quality measures to Medicare and commercial payers.

Orlando Health is depending on its population health management vendor to do the heavy lifting, including data integration and work-flow assessments, data mapping to protocols, system configuration, training, and implementation. The vendor is also identifying and addressing problems with data integrity, including those that originate in the clinical work flow. The organization would prefer not to rely solely on health plans' claims data because they are usually not timely enough to be actionable.

An early win for Orlando Health has been its use of the vendor's patient-outreach program. This ongoing automated messaging campaign has persuaded many patients who need preventive or chronic care to make appointments with their doctors. Orlando Health has also used it as the basis for a local school system's campaign to increase the use of breast cancer screening. Many women are now getting mammograms as a result.

In addition, Orlando Health is using an automated care-management program to identify care gaps and intervene with patients who have hypertension, high cholesterol, or diabetes. It employs a different form of outreach provided by the same firm to follow up with patients after hospital and ED discharges. The next step will be to integrate these tools with a single patient portal for the CIN.

For Orlando Health, automation is the key to both clinical integration and population health management. By automatically risk-stratifying the population, identifying care gaps, engaging patients, managing care for high-risk patients, and evaluating performance, Orlando Health can quickly scale up its CIN without spending a huge amount of money on care coordination and care management.

Case Study: Jackson Health Network

The Jackson Health Network (JHN) is a clinically integrated network in Jackson, Michigan. Affiliated with Allegiance Health, JHN includes 75 percent of the local physicians, including 218 employed and independent doctors in twenty-eight specialties. The CIN was formed to improve community health and to enable the area physicians—most of whom are in small practices—to negotiate value-based contracts with payers.

Several factors have aided JHN on its road to clinical integration. First, 60 percent of its primary care practices have been recognized as patient-centered medical homes. Second, more than 150 JHN physicians, including employed and community doctors, are using the same electronic health record, which was subsidized by Allegiance. Third, the county health department is using that EHR, too, and is aligned with JHN's health-improvement goals. And fourth, the CIN is using a suite of automated tools designed for population health management, including automated patient outreach.

JHN now has a web-based patient registry that it has aligned with its case-management information system. Analytics applied to the registry enable JHN to risk-stratify its population. A quality-reporting system based on the same registry is enabling physicians to see how they compare with their peers and to identify the care gaps of individual patients. Each specialty has its own report card, which is used to determine incentive payments to physicians.

JHN discovered that its physicians were reporting on 600 metrics to various parties. The CIN has cut that down to seventy measures that all of its physicians are committed to using. But it's still finding it difficult to get all the local health plans to use the same set of metrics.

JHN has subsequently planned to get its specialists more involved in clinical integration. It will also pilot care-management programs and expand work-flow redesign in its practices.

Like every other CIN and accountable care organization, JHN has had to work hard to clean up its data and preserve data integrity. The use of a common EHR and the ability to maintain a single version by updating it for all users has helped. So has the prevalence of pay-for-performance in Michigan, which has accustomed physicians to entering the required data in their EHRs. But they don't always enter the information in the right fields, and JHN has encountered difficulties in importing data from labs and imaging centers outside of the CIN. In addition, there are the customary problems with patient identification and provider attribution.

Nevertheless, JHN's managers are fairly confident that they've worked through these challenges, and they are up and running with their new care-management solution. They are also expanding work-flow redesign and trying to get specialists more involved in the clinically integrated network.

Five Ways to Leverage Predictive Modeling for Population Health Management

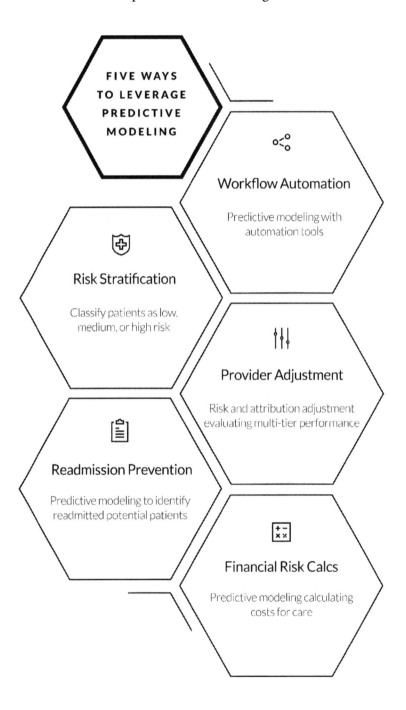

Chapter 6

Predictive Modeling

- *Introduction*: The front end of the infrastructure for population health management is predictive modeling, which forecasts which patients are likely to get sick or sicker in the near term. Predictive analytics should be combined with automation tools to help care teams improve outcomes and lower costs. It can also be used to help organizations manage financial risk.
- *Background*: Predictive modeling can be used for risk stratification of a population or risk adjustment. The approach, which grew out of health plans' actuarial predictions, is now being applied by health-care organizations to manage care and avoid readmissions. Health forecasting has limits, some of which are related to many organizations' inability to translate it into action.
- *Turning predictions into action*: Both predictive modeling tools from health plans and the applications built into some EHRs use claims data. To make health forecasting actionable, it should be based to a greater extent on clinical data that are as current as possible.
- *Risk stratification*: Risk stratification is used to classify the population into high-, medium-, and low-risk categories so care teams can deliver appropriate interventions to each group. It can also be refined to prioritize those high-risk patients who need help immediately. And it can enable care teams to address the needs of those most likely to become sick or sicker.

- *Provider attribution/risk adjustment*: Correct provider attribution for patients is necessary for care coordination and performance measurement. Risk adjustment, which is used in measuring performance and negotiating contracts, uses different inputs than other kinds of predictive modeling.

- *Financial risk*: Predictive modeling is key to calculating the financial impact of a risk contract on an organization. While the positive predictive value of these applications varies for hospital and ED admissions, it's possible to predict with a fair degree of accuracy the likelihood that a particular patient will generate high costs.

- *Data sources*: The more data you have, the better you will be able to predict outcomes. But every data source available today has shortcomings. Claims data are neither timely nor precise; clinical data are usually limited to a single organization; and patient-reported data, except for patient-satisfaction surveys, are largely missing.

As the health-care industry continues its transition to new care-delivery and payment models, an increasing number of health-care organizations are embracing population health management (see chapter 1). By helping people manage their own health so that they need less health care and by proactively managing the care of chronically ill patients, these organizations seek to achieve the Triple Aim of improving the quality of care, reducing health costs, and enhancing the patient experience.

To manage population health, health-care systems and group practices must build the requisite infrastructure, including software tools designed for data analysis and work-flow automation. The front end of this IT infrastructure is a type of analytic solution known variously as predictive analytics, predictive modeling, or health forecasting. In a population heath management context, these algorithmic tools predict which people are likely to get sick or sicker in the near term.

This is crucially important information to provider organizations and health plans that take financial responsibility for care. Ten percent of patients generate roughly 70 percent of health costs; 5 percent account for half of health outlays.[1,2] By identifying which people are high risk or likely to become high risk, risk-bearing entities can intervene with them to improve their outcomes and lower health costs.

Most health plans offer case management, disease management, and health-coaching programs to these members. Some health-care organizations seek to ensure that high-risk patients receive necessary services and day-to-day support from care managers. To improve outcomes and lower costs, these organizations must connect predictive analytics with work-flow automation tools that enable care teams to intervene with the right patients at the right time in the right way.

In this chapter, we explain what predictive modeling is and what it can and can't do. We show how health-care organizations can make the insights of predictive modeling actionable for financial managers and clinical teams. We provide examples of how predictive analytics, population risk stratification, and risk adjustment are applied in practice. We also review the kinds of data required to do predictive modeling and compare the value of each data source for taking action.

Background

Predictive modeling is a branch of clinical and business intelligence (C&BI) that is used to forecast the future health status of individuals and to classify patients by their current health risk (risk stratification). It can also be used in risk adjustment to compare the aggregate health risks of one physician's or one organization's patients to those of another doctor or health-care entity. Most important from the viewpoint of health-care organizations that assume financial risk for care, predictive analytics can be employed to predict health costs for individuals and populations.

Predictive analytics depend on computer algorithms that can recognize patterns in data. The applications draw inferences from the data about the likelihood of patients developing certain conditions or exacerbations of their existing conditions. In some cases, the developers of predictive analytics use large public databases as the basis of their models. Other models are built with data about specific patient populations.

To create a predictive algorithm, developers define a problem, then select and evaluate models to solve it. After selecting the best model and validating it, they test it by applying it to a real-world database. They may also improve the accuracy of the predictive tool by using known outcomes to "train" the algorithm.

Health plans have been doing predictive modeling for years, using paid claims data. The precursor of this approach is insurance underwriting, in which actuaries identify insurance applicants who are likely to generate high costs and calculate how much to charge individuals and employers for coverage. Over the past decade, health plans have also used their information on patients' health risks to identify those who might benefit from disease and case-management programs. Because of the rapid turnover in their membership, most plans have limited the focus of these programs to the sickest people to ensure a return on investment.

Few health-care organizations did any health forecasting until the emergence of accountable care organizations and new payment models that put them at financial risk. The majority of health-care systems still don't have the enterprise data warehouses or registries required for this approach.[3] Those that do are more likely to use these databases for retrospective review than for predictive modeling.[4] But that's expected to change in the next few years as more organizations take on financial risk for care.

Another factor that is currently driving the uptake of predictive analytics is the financial penalties that hospitals incur if they readmit too many Medicare patients. Not surprisingly, a number of vendors offer applications designed to predict which patients are most likely to be readmitted. At the same time, studies of predictive analytics related to readmissions have proliferated.

Some of these readmission tools appear to be moderately accurate.[5,6] In addition, a predictive modeling application that calculates the odds of a patient developing a serious chronic condition or having a heart attack has been shown to be effective.[7] Nevertheless, a recent paper on health forecasting points out:

> There is little evidence regarding how or whether forecasting improves healthcare value. This is due to both the modest level of research and what is termed the "impactibility" problem. That is, even if prediction algorithms accurately identify at-risk patients, intervening to achieve desired outcomes is often inhibited by limitations of current disease management approaches or the general state of medical science.[8]

To put it another way, fairly few organizations are using the insights of predictive modeling effectively to improve chronic disease care. But that is bound to change. While financial forecasting and readmission prevention currently drive the use of predictive modeling in health care, the most important use of this approach will be in population health management, because chronic diseases account for 75 percent of health costs.[9] Indeed, a recent study of Medicare data shows that improving care for patients with complex diseases is the most effective way to "bend the cost curve."[10] Therefore, the "consumers" of predictive analytics tools will expand from the CFOs to the frontline physicians and other care-team members.

Turning predictions into action

Predictive analytics are worthless unless their insights prompt actions. In the area of population health management, these actions include alerts to providers at the point of care and information that enables care managers to prioritize their patient interventions. On the financial side, health-care organizations can use predictive modeling to forecast the cost of care delivery so they can evaluate risk contracts.

To be valuable in care management, predictive analytics must be timely. Claims data are necessary to predict the annual costs of caring for a patient population, but information that is three months old will not help clinicians intervene with patients to improve their outcomes. For that, organizations need the latest progress notes, lab results, and medications for a patient—in other words, the clinical data in an EHR. When these clinical data are combined with patient-reported data between visits, the information available for analytics is even more up-to-date.

Some EHR vendors offer predictive analytics that are capable of doing risk stratification. These analytics modules use claims data, rather than EHR data.[11] Claims data can be used for this task because risk stratification at the broadest level does not require near-real-time data. But clinical information is required to predict health status accurately enough to design cost-effective interventions. Moreover, claims data reflect prior care events and patterns but don't capture recent changes in health behavior; for instance, a heart attack survivor may now be exercising, eating right, and no longer smoking.[12]

Risk stratification

Predictive modeling forms the basis of risk stratification, which is used to identify the patients who will generate the majority of costs in the near future. Populations can be classified into high-, medium-, and low-risk patients with a fair degree of confidence. Depending on which of those categories a patient is slotted into, he or she might receive intensive care management, online education and support in managing his or her own care so that chronic conditions don't worsen, or just education and encouragement in maintaining a healthy lifestyle.

To prevent people from becoming high-risk, it is essential to keep track of and support those who are healthy today but could become sick tomorrow. Of the patients who generate the highest costs in a given year, only 30 percent had high costs a year earlier.[13]

At a population level, organizations can use risk stratification to decide how best to direct their resources. For the large number of patients who are obese and have high blood pressure, for example, organizations might decide to drill down further to identify patients within this group who have other chronic conditions and unhealthy behaviors that would increase the risk of an acute event.

With this kind of refined data set, organizations can tailor care-team alerts and patient interventions by risk cohort. Providers can use care alerts to make sure that that the most urgent problems of patients are addressed during office visits. Other clinical staffers can use the insights of predictive analytics to reach out to patients who need to be seen. Care managers can be prompted to intervene with certain patients and can also design campaigns to provide assistance to people with less-urgent needs. For example, they might decide that group visits with an endocrinologist would be helpful to patients with diabetes who have not been able to lower their HbA1c levels.

At a population-wide level, this kind of work is very time-consuming and labor-intensive. To make effective use of predictive analytics, health-care organizations should couple these applications with tools that automate the work flow of care teams. For example, predictive analytics can be applied to electronic registries to give care managers the tools they need to intervene with patients based on their health status. High-risk patients and other patients with care gaps who have not seen their providers recently can be contacted via automated messaging.

Automation can help organizations manage the majority of patients, because most people are healthy or have moderate chronic conditions that don't require intensive care management. But it is crucially important to identify those patients who are not yet very sick but may move into the high-risk category within the next year. By helping to ensure they follow their providers' care plans and by engaging them in managing their own health, care teams can help to reduce the number of these people who become seriously ill.

Predictive modeling is also required to identify those who are already high-risk and to prioritize those who need help right away. The sickest patients, such as those with metastatic cancer, HIV, and end-stage renal disease, will automatically go into care-management programs. Risk stratification can help identify others who could likely benefit from care management, based on rules such as their number of diagnoses, types and numbers of medications, and prior hospital admissions. But in a large population, thousands of patients might fit these definitions—far too many for care managers to handle personally with limited resources. So it may be necessary to use criteria such as prior costs from claims data and clinical risk status to further prioritize which patients need immediate attention.

Another key point is that there is a direct correlation between comorbidities and health risk. In 2010, for example, Medicare beneficiaries with multiple conditions accounted for nearly all readmissions. Average annual spending for Medicare patients with six or more conditions was $32,658, versus $12,174 for people with four or five conditions; $5,698 for those with two or three diseases; and $2,025 for people with one or no conditions. So a good predictive analytics tool must factor in those comorbidities.[14]

Clinical judgment and culture

When it comes to individual patients, predictive algorithms cannot predict who will be hospitalized or who will need to visit the ER with a high degree of accuracy. So the findings of predictive tools must be combined with clinical judgment to produce the best results in most cases.

For example, predictive modeling might indicate that an elderly patient who leaves the hospital with several conditions and is on multiple medications is a prime candidate for readmission. But one patient who has those risk factors might receive good home health care and be cognitively alert, whereas another with the same risk factors might have no support at home and might have little ability to understand discharge instructions. A physician who knows those two patients will be able to tell which of them is at higher risk of readmission.

To be of any use in improving the quality of care, predictive modeling tools must be accepted by clinicians. That requires some cultural change on the part of physicians who don't want to take advice from a computer. Here again, the role of clinical judgment is paramount: If doctors believe that their judgment is being overridden by a computer algorithm, they'll rebel; but if they view predictive analytics as a kind of clinical decision support, they'll be more likely to use this tool, much as they use drug-interaction checks in e-prescribing applications to avoid medication errors.

Provider attribution/risk adjustment

A prerequisite of population health management is the correct matching of patients to their primary providers. Accurate provider attribution is required for both risk stratification and risk adjustment, which is used in comparing the performance of organizations and individual providers. Asaf Bitton, MD, a researcher at Harvard Medical School's Center for Primary Care, explains that attribution takes effort but can be done properly:

> Attribution happens with about 60–90 percent fidelity, so some patients fall through the cracks. It is a key starting point for knowing generally who your clinicians care for, and getting to near-100 percent attribution within your EHR is an important milestone at the outset of your journey toward population management.[15]

Risk adjustment enables payers and provider organizations to compare the performance of clinicians, practices, or hospitals fairly by differentiating between the characteristics of the patients they serve.

The most common type of risk adjustor is based on the severity of the health conditions in a particular population. The ACG Predictive Model from Johns Hopkins University, for example, is widely used in provider profiling. Based on diagnosis and pharmacy data, it describes the differences between providers' case mixes.[16] Verisk offers another commercial risk adjustor that's closely related to the one used by Medicare and the new state health insurance exchanges. Its DxCG risk adjustor uses Diagnostic Cost Groups and RxGroups. Like the ACG predictive model, DxCG depends on claims data.

The difference between risk adjustment and the broader kind of predictive modeling lies in the data inputs. Whereas both approaches use diagnostic codes, for example, risk adjustment excludes prior costs and utilization of services, which might reward inefficient providers. Predictive analytics, on the other hand, embraces prior costs and a wide range of other variables that might play a role in future health outcomes and utilization of resources.

Financial risk

Beyond measuring the efficiency of individual providers, health-care organizations that aspire to take financial risk must be able to project the costs that their patient population is likely to generate. Predictive analytics can be a big help to these organizations, but they must also recognize the limitations of these tools.

Take hospital admissions, which account for a large portion of health costs. The positive predictive value of a predictive modeling application might be as high as 80 percent, but only for high-risk patients. Applied to people with moderate health risks, the same predictor might have a lower positive predictive value. Predictive analytics can forecast which patients will go to the ER with good accuracy in some cases. But because of the unpredictable nature of some ER visits, which may be related to car accidents or various types of trauma, the software doesn't predict ER visits as well as hospitalizations.[17]

However, it is possible to gauge the likelihood that a particular patient will generate high costs in the following year. To calculate that probability, an organization must have data on a variety of risk factors, including information on the individual's prior costs and utilization of services, current health status, diagnoses, lab results, and medications; it would also help to know something about the nonclinical factors that are discussed below. Applying an algorithm to those variables yields a risk score for each patient, based on their individual characteristics, and an average score can be computed from that.

The organization benchmarks its average risk score against national standards or its historical costs. If its average cost to care for a patient is $1,000 per year, for example, it multiplies that amount times the number of patients and their average risk score to predict what it will spend in the next year. The organization can then decide whether the capitation payment it's being offered is sufficient to cover its expected costs.

Each risk contract that an organization negotiates covers a separate population, comprised of patients that are covered by a particular health plan. So providers may have to use the predictive modeling approach described above multiple times for each payer from which they are planning to take capitation. (Payment bundling, while it also involves risk, requires different calculations based on episodes of care.)

The health risks of individuals are always changing, of course, and a few "outliers" could have catastrophic costs in the next year. Large organizations have a better ability to withstand the financial consequences of these catastrophes than small ones do. But no provider organization should take on financial risk without stop-loss insurance to cushion it against these unexpected losses.

Predictive modeling can help organizations factor in these outliers and prevent at least some of them from racking up huge expenses. By tracking catastrophic cases over time, an organization can get a sense of which patients are likely to hit the stop-loss limit, which might be $100,000. It can then provide extra resources to ensure those patients receive appropriate care. While it's impossible to forecast all catastrophic events, focusing intensively on those that are most likely to occur can have strongly positive results for both the patients and the bottom line.

Data sources

To do predictive modeling, organizations must have access to multiple sources of data that describe the health status of individuals and populations as completely and as currently as possible. The information must be very timely to be actionable for care management.

"The more data you have, the better able you are to predict outcomes," Patrick Gordon, executive director of the Colorado Beacon Consortium, said recently. "Access to more actionable data within a process driven by clinical judgment and shared patient decision-making improves the ability of a practice team to proactively align resources with patient needs."[18]

Nevertheless, the data available for predictive modeling today have some serious deficiencies. Claims data are neither timely nor precise; clinical data are usually limited to a single organization; and patient-reported data, except for patient-satisfaction surveys, are largely missing. Until the information that health-care organizations can apply to predictive modeling improves, it will be more useful for some purposes, such as risk stratification of populations, than for others, such as predicting the health risks of individuals with a high degree of accuracy.

Some health-care systems are beginning to combine claims and clinical data in ways that enable them to use predictive analytics more effectively. And as risk-bearing organizations seek to engage patients in their own care, they are beginning to recognize the importance of patient-reported data.

Claims data

Claims data usually lag the provision of services by one to three months, but they offer the broadest view of the health-care services that patients have received and the prescriptions they've filled. In the view of Jonathan Weiner, a professor of health policy at Johns Hopkins University, accountable care organizations (ACOs) and other entities that manage population health will be heavily dependent on claims data for the next decade or longer.[19]

For purposes of calculating the financial costs and risks of a particular patient population, there is no substitute for claims information. The clinical data available to a health-care organization are generally limited to the care provided within that enterprise, but everybody who provides services to insured patients submits claims.

Some health plans make claims data available to providers and ACOs. Other health-care organizations that are self-insured employers have begun the journey toward population health management by using the claims data for their own employees. But unless an organization includes a health plan—such as Kaiser Permanente, HealthPartners, or Geisinger—it is unlikely to have access to complete claims or encounter data for most or all of its patient population.

The analytic tools now available to health-care providers are mainly those that insurers have historically applied to claims. Today, when clinical data are combined with claims, they must be integrated into that framework. But eventually, the approach to predictive modeling will become more clinically oriented, and claims data will be used to round out the picture.

Clinical data

The spread of electronic health records in recent years has led to a massive growth in the amount of digitized clinical data. But much of these data are unstructured, making them unavailable to predictive modeling and other analytic tools. Moreover, because patients receive health care from multiple providers, clinical data generated by one organization may not be sufficient to describe what has happened to a patient or that person's current health status. Health information exchange is improving, but still has a long way to go.

According to an HIMSS Analytics white paper on analytics, the data challenges to health-care organizations include:

- getting data into the system in a structured way, whether they're collected on paper or come from another source, such as prescription fill data from pharmacies;
- issues with extracting data from source formats and combining them into a usable aggregated database; and
- missing data elements required for analysis. In some cases, this occurs because providers fail to enter data in the correct fields. Data may also be unobtainable if providers cannot exchange information electronically or if the data are housed in multiple databases within an enterprise.[20]

Even if an organization has an enterprise data warehouse, it might find that it takes too long to aggregate and normalize the data for the predictive analytics that are used in care management. A health-care system might solve this problem by building a registry within the warehouse and making sure that the registry receives updates on clinical data, such as lab results, within twenty-four hours of them becoming available. In an organization that includes multiple inpatient and ambulatory EHRs, one solution is to create a registry that receives data directly from the organization's or ACO's internal health information exchange.[21]

Patient-reported data

To increase the accuracy of predictive analytics and risk stratification, it is essential to obtain information on how patients regard their own health status, their nonclinical risk factors, including health behavior, and their obstacles to managing their own health. Some of this data can be collected during visits to their providers, but much of it changes continually and must be gathered between visits or after discharge from the hospital. Consequently, organizations must provide ways for patients to report this data themselves on a regular basis.

The importance of patient-reported data cannot be overestimated. For example, a particular patient might be considered at moderate risk based on clinical data such as slightly elevated blood pressure and obesity. But that patient's propensity to become seriously ill is much greater if one considers his or her lifestyle, socioeconomic status, and ability to obtain healthy food. The chance of a recently discharged patient being readmitted, similarly, will be higher if that person has no one to take care of him or her at home, is depressed, and can't afford the copayments for prescription drugs.

Among the types of patient surveys that have been developed for collecting information pertinent to health risks are health risk assessments (HRAs), patient activation surveys, and functional status surveys. HRAs, which are used mostly by large, self-insured employers, ask people about a wide range of health and lifestyle factors. Activation instruments measure a patient's knowledge, skills, and confidence in managing his or her own health care. Functional status surveys, which some providers use to measure outcomes after hospitalizations or post-acute care, ask patients how they're feeling and how well they're functioning. Both generic and condition-specific instruments are available for this purpose.[22]

The use of patient-reported data in predictive modeling is rare today. But the Cincinnati Beacon Community—one of seventeen around the country that are funded by the government to explore the frontiers of health IT—has used HRAs to help hospitals reduce readmissions.[23] Some hospitals and rehabilitation facilities use functional status surveys, but the data from them are not being entered in EHRs.

Five Ways to Leverage Predictive Modeling

1. *Risk stratification.* Classify patients as low-, medium-, or high-risk. Use that information to allocate resources at a population-wide level, identify high-risk patients, alert providers and care managers about those patients, and design interventions to prevent other people from becoming high-risk.

2. *Work-flow automation.* Couple predictive modeling with automation tools that enable providers to reach out to patients with care gaps and allow care managers to touch more patients in various ways, ranging from high-touch case management to web-based education and coaching.

3. *Readmission prevention.* Use preventive modeling to identify which patients are most likely to be readmitted. Intervene with these patients so they receive the support they need to avoid readmission.

4. *Provider attribution and risk adjustment.* Apply risk adjustment to evaluate the performance of individual providers, sites, and your whole organization in comparison to others. Use risk adjustment to measure variations in care, improve quality, and show payers how your organization ranks in utilization and quality.

5. *Financial risk calculations.* Employ predictive modeling to calculate how much care delivery will likely cost for your population in the coming year. Use these figures to determine whether the organization will lose or make money under proposed risk contracts.

Conclusion

Predictive analytics are emerging as must-have tools for any organization that wants to do population health management. These analytics cover a wide range of applications, including those that forecast patients' future health, classify them by their current health status, predict hospitalizations and readmissions, and adjust providers' performance evaluations by their case mix. In addition, predictive modeling is being used extensively to help organizations calculate the likely cost of caring for a particular population. This is an increasingly important function as more and more organizations take financial risk for care.

Predictive modeling has some serious limitations. The biggest challenges have to do with the available data. Claims and clinical data each have their own issues, and patient-reported data—which could form a much fuller picture of a patient's situation—are largely missing. But predictive analytics are already invaluable tools in the new health-care delivery models. As the data improve and new algorithms are devised, their value will increase further, but only if they're connected to work-flow automation solutions that make their insights actionable.

Predictive analytics, as discussed above, are as important to managing within a budget as they are to producing better patient outcomes and improving an organization's quality scores. But along with other population health management IT solutions, they don't fit comfortably into traditional notions of return on investment, because they're not designed to increase revenues. As we discuss in the next chapter, organizations need to change their definition of ROI as they move into the era of value-based reimbursement.

Three Sources of Population Health ROI
(Example using a 200 provider organization)

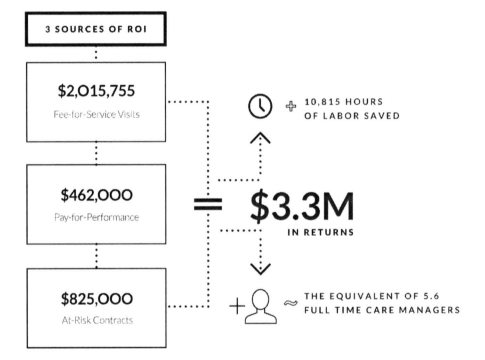

Chapter 7

Automation Solutions and the ROI of Change

- *Introduction*: Organizations can achieve ROI in a value-based reimbursement environment.
- *Background*: As financial pressures increase on health-care organizations, new payment models require a different kind of health IT infrastructure.
- *The new return on investment*: ROI from population health management IT, based on improved quality and efficiency, is becoming important with the emergence of new health-care payment models.
- *Automated population health management*: Automation tools can manage population health, avoiding manual methods that are expensive and time-consuming.
- *How automation produces ROI*: Patient outreach, analytics, care management, patient engagement, and transitions of care can all be performed efficiently at a population-wide level with the help of automation and analytic solutions.
- *How to calculate ROI*: The ROI from using three automation tools is calculated for a hypothetical group of 200 physicians.

As the US health-care system begins to shift toward a value-based reimbursement model, health-care organizations need to adjust their thinking about the concept of return on investment.

Conventional ROI measures the ratio between the cost of new equipment, software, or staff and the savings or revenues they generate. But in a world where providers are rewarded for meeting quality targets or are at financial risk for medical costs, the definition of ROI has to change. It should reflect the ability of solutions to increase staff efficiency and contain health-care costs.

Analytic and automation tools can be used to manage population health, and they're now indispensable in helping providers obtain higher value-based payments. The best technological solutions designed for population health management offer four types of ROI:

- medical cost savings that increase provider revenue under risk contracts
- bigger pay for performance rewards because of patient outreach and higher-quality care
- increased fee-for-service revenues from patient visits to fill care gaps
- operational savings that can be reinvested in care management

What follows is a discussion of how health-care organizations should measure health IT ROI in the new environment. Examples of how specific health-care providers approach this issue are included. The chapter concludes with a hypothetical scenario that shows how ROI can be calculated.

Background

Hospitals and health-care organizations face an increasingly adverse financial environment. Hospital margins returned to prerecession levels in 2012, mainly because of increased emergency department and outpatient business.[1] But health-care reform and value-based reimbursement are creating new challenges.

The Affordable Care Act (ACA) has proved to be a mixed blessing for health-care organizations so far. Fewer of the uninsured are signing up for coverage than expected.[2] Only about half of the states have expanded Medicaid.[3] High deductibles in many insurance exchange plans are expected to discourage some members from seeking care.[4] And some insurance companies are keeping costs down in the exchange plans by selectively contracting with lower-cost providers.[5]

Meanwhile, Medicare and Medicaid payments continue to cover only part of care-delivery costs.[6] The percentage of hospital expenses that go to bad debt and charity care is rising.[7] And the ability of hospitals to bargain with commercial payers depends largely on their market clout—a key reason for the new wave of consolidation among health-care providers.[8] Physicians have little bargaining power: their average reimbursement from private plans fell 9 percent in 2012 and 10 percent in 2011.[9]

Health-care organizations also must bear growing costs that result from unfunded government mandates. These include investments in health IT to meet Meaningful Use requirements that, for hospitals and large physician practices, can be in the multimillion-dollar range.[10] The industry-wide conversion to ICD-10 diagnostic codes will also be very expensive when software and training costs and productivity losses are included.[11]

Hospitals have absorbed $113 billion in legislative and regulatory payment cuts since 2010.[12] The Centers for Medicare and Medicaid Services (CMS) is also reducing payments to hospitals that have excessive readmission rates.[13] Many hospitals are being penalized financially under Medicare's value-based payment program if their costs are too high or if they miss quality targets.[14] Starting next year, groups of one hundred or more eligible professionals will be subject to CMS's value-based modifier.[15]

Transition to value-based payments

The introduction of the value-based modifier is part of a larger trend in the industry: the move to value-based reimbursement. While fee-for-service still dominates, health-care providers can expect to see value-based payment methods account for a progressively larger amount of their revenue in coming years.

Value-based reimbursement started fifteen years ago with the introduction of pay-for-performance programs. Under these programs, health plans offer financial incentives to physicians for meeting their targets on a number of quality measures.[16] To reach these targets, practices must regularly measure their performance—a nearly impossible task without the use of information technology.

Several years ago, the patient-centered medical home (PCMH) movement began to gain traction. As payers started to see the potential of this approach for lowering costs, they began to reward physician practices for gaining PCMH recognition. The National Committee on Quality Assurance (NCQA), which recognizes the bulk of medical homes, requires that practices show 26 elements in six categories for the highest level of PCMH recognition. The majority of those criteria involve the use of health IT in one way or another.[17]

Meanwhile, both CMS and private payers are encouraging the development of accountable care organizations (ACOs), networks of hospitals and practices that take responsibility for the cost and quality of care. From 2012 to 2013, the number of ACOs doubled, and it now exceeds 600 organizations.[18,19] Some ACOs participate in the Medicare Shared Savings Program (MSSP), which allows them to either share savings only or to take financial risk from CMS.[20] Many ACOs have shared-savings or risk contracts with commercial insurers, some of which are also ACO codevelopers.[21]

The MSSP requires ACOs to meet quality goals on thirty-three measures.[22] Because of this and because they must coordinate care among disparate providers, ACOs are heavily dependent on health IT. As we explain later, they must also use specialized solutions to manage population health, which is especially important if they're taking risk.

Bundled payments, which are budgets for episodes of care, are also growing in importance. CMS recently launched a bundled-payment demonstration project,[23] and many health-care organizations are entering or considering entering bundled-payment agreements with private payers.[24] Typically, these arrangements involve a hospitalization and post-acute care for a specified period, although some providers are also experimenting with payment bundling for episodes of chronic care. Again, health IT is indispensable, not only for communications between hospitals and other providers, but also for tracking services and dividing payments.

At this point, most health-care organizations recognize that the payment system is changing and that they must prepare for value-based reimbursement. They know they can't do it without health IT. But in the current economic climate, they must be sure that they will see a return on their investment in software. So their financial officers ask, "How do we measure ROI?" The answer depends on the kinds of IT tools they acquire and how those tools can help them achieve their strategic goals.

The new return on investment

The evidence of "hard" ROI from legacy health-care IT is mixed,[25,26] and the "soft" return from quality improvement has been difficult to prove. But when new applications for population health management (PHM) are combined with existing clinical data, the case that health IT can generate ROI is much stronger.

Today's clinical applications are typically designed for traditional fee-for-service sick care, not for PHM.[27] For a practice to become a patient-centered medical home or function effectively within an ACO, or for a health-care organization to form a well-coordinated, high-quality ACO, it needs ancillary applications that can use clinical and claims data to manage population health. By automating the process of ensuring that all patients receive the right care at the right time, these tools can help organizations increase their value-based reimbursement, thereby achieving ROI.

Even in a fee-for-service environment, some ROI can be expected from the use of patient-outreach applications that spur patients to make appointments for needed preventive and chronic care. But most of the ROI from PHM solutions emerges in the business models that reward higher quality and efficiency. These rewards include pay-for-performance (P4P) incentives, patient-centered medical home payments, ACO shared-savings and risk contracts, bundled payments, and the potential upside of Medicare's value-based modifiers.

According to the Health Information Management and Systems Society (HIMSS), health IT can create five kinds of value, including:

- *satisfaction* of patients, providers, staff, and others;
- *treatment/clinical*—patient safety, quality of care, and efficiency;
- *electronic information/data*—use of evidence-based guidelines, data sharing, population health, and quality reporting;
- *prevention/patient education*—improved disease surveillance and patient compliance with therapies; and
- *savings* from improvements such as reduced days in accounts receivable, patient wait times, and emergency-department admissions.[28]

In HIMSS's schema, value extends far beyond the hard ROI of immediate savings and revenue increases. The value created by health IT benefits not only providers, but also patients, payers, and the community—in other words, those who determine what providers are worth and what they should be paid. If value-based reimbursement is framed in these terms, PHM solutions hold the key to ROI in the new health-care environment.

Automated population health management

Population health management requires health-care organizations to optimize the health of their patients. Instead of focusing mainly on diagnosis and treatment, providers must also try to prevent patients from getting sick or sicker. They must do this as efficiently as possible to conserve the limited amount of health-care resources.

The Population Health Alliance defines PHM as an approach to care delivery that includes these components:

- the central care delivery and leadership roles of the primary care physician;
- an emphasis on patient activation, involvement, and personal responsibility; and
- the patient focus and capacity expansion of care coordination provided through wellness, disease, and chronic care-management programs.[29]

To manage population health, a provider organization must ensure that all of its patients receive appropriate preventive and chronic care. Since not all patients visit their providers on a timely basis or adhere to their care plans, organizations engaged in PHM have to reach out to noncompliant patients between visits. They must also monitor their patients' health, engage them in self-care, and give them educational materials about their conditions. They have to stratify their populations by health risk and provide care management to their highest-risk patients. And they must supply clinical decision support to their providers so that they know which patients need preventive or chronic care when they come to the office.

It is too expensive and time-consuming for any health-care organization to do all of this work manually. For example, many organizations have hired care managers to manage severely ill patients. These care managers may not be able to serve all the people who need their help because they must spend so much time doing routine tasks like searching for patient data and trying to contact patients.

The addition of care managers and other health professionals required to do population health management substantially increases the ratio of clinical staff to physicians in patient-centered medical homes. In a 2013 study, researchers interviewed nine administrators of primary care practices, seven of which included at least one PCMH. Based on the results of those interviews and other data, they calculated that a PCMH requires 4.25 FTE staff members per FTE physician, 1.57 staffers more than the average primary care doctor does in a non-PCMH practice. Most of this difference represents the hiring of nurse care managers. The incremental cost of this proposed infrastructure is $4.68 per member per month.[30]

Health-care systems and group practices can't afford this many care managers, so they must consider ways to automate the process. Based on time-motion studies at Prevea Health, a multispecialty group in Green Bay, Wisconsin, automation enables care managers to manage two to three times as many patients as they can with manual methods. Routine tasks such as chart prep and patient follow-up communications take less time when they're automated, the internal studies show.

Automation software can enable organizations to reach the entire patient population on a periodic or as-needed basis, whether or not patients seek care. It can provide care managers with near-real-time information on patient health needs that allows them to prioritize their interventions. And it can provide timely alerts to providers about patient care gaps so they can be addressed during office visits.

The ROI of automation tools comes from multiple sources. Among other things, these applications can be used to:

- message patients to make office appointments for necessary care;
- streamline operations, reducing the cost of labor;
- enable care managers to work with additional patients;
- improve the patient experience, helping organizations retain patients and increase market share; and
- improve health-care quality and reduce costs, enabling providers to qualify for higher value-based reimbursement.

The literature on the ROI of these automation tools is slim. However, there is evidence that the patient-centered medical home (PCMH)— which relies on health IT as the basis of care coordination and quality improvement—has helped some health-care organizations cut the cost of care. For example:

- Blue Cross Blue Shield of Michigan found that practices with full PCMH implementation had savings of $26.37 per member per month.
- In the Military Health System, the PCMH model led to 6.8 percent fewer ED visits, a 13 percent reduction in pharmacy costs, and a 16 percent decrease in ancillary costs.
- At UPMC Health Plan in Pennsylvania, a PCMH pilot was associated with 5.1 percent fewer ED visits; a smaller increase in hospitalizations than non-PCMH practices; 12.5 percent fewer readmissions; and a 160 percent return on investment.
- CareFirst BlueCross Blue Shield of Maryland saved $98 million on its PCMH initiative.[31]

Where provider organizations participate in shared-savings programs, part of these savings goes back to them. The initial progress report of the Medicare Shared Savings Program shows that these gains are real for some accountable care organizations. In the first year of the MSSP, savings exceeded $380 million, and nearly half of the participating ACOs had lower expenditures than predicted. Of those fifty-four ACOs, twenty-nine generated $128 million in savings that they shared with Medicare.[32]

How automation produces ROI

Technology-driven automation makes PHM cost-effective by reducing the amount of work required to care continuously for a patient population. Among the areas where automation is recommended are patient outreach, analytics, care management, patient engagement and transitions of care. Here's a brief summary of each.

Patient outreach

Population health management requires a health-care organization to maintain regular contact with all of its patients, whether or not they visit their providers. To do this kind of outreach efficiently and in a way that results in better health outcomes, organizations need several kinds of automation tools. First, they must have patient registries that list all patients, their health problems, and what has been done for them. Combined with software that stratifies the patients by health risk and that shows their care gaps, these registries can be used to trigger automated messaging to patients who need preventive or chronic care.

Research has shown that these kinds of outreach programs raise the percentage of patients who visit doctors to obtain the recommended care. Besides improving the health of the population—which can garner value-based incentives—such tools also drive increases in fee-for-service revenue when patients visit their providers.

Prevea Health, a 180-physician multispecialty group in Green Bay, Wisconsin, has made good use of these tools. Since 2009, Prevea has built patient-centered medical homes in fifteen primary care sites that include fifty providers and seventeen care managers who care for 29,000 patients. But the group found that its medical homes couldn't manage population health effectively without automation.

Prevea automated the processes of identifying gaps in care and performing patient outreach. Patients who needed care received automated messages asking them to make appointments to see their providers. As a result, appointments for preventive and chronic care soared. According to a peer-reviewed study, patients with diabetes who received automated messages were three times as likely to visit their physicians and have an HbA1c test as noncontacted patients. And twice as many patients with hypertension who received this intervention had both a visit and a systolic blood pressure reading recorded in Prevea's EHR.[33]

Prevea hasn't done a formal analysis of its ROI from using automated outreach to bring in additional patients for follow-up care. But Bon Secours Virginia Medical Group did such a study and found that automated messaging generated $7 million in revenues from follow-up visits. Those 40,000 visits created an ROI of 16:1 on the group's technology investment, according to a Phytel case study.

Analytics

To use health IT in population health management, an organization must first develop the capability to collect, aggregate, and normalize the data on its patient population. After it has accomplished that task, it needs analytic and other tools to make the information actionable. Among these tools are applications for risk stratification, care-gap identification, care planning, and care management. These solutions can be used for multiple purposes, including automated patient messaging, alerting providers, setting priorities for care managers, engaging patients, and evaluating provider and organizational performance.

Bon Secours Virginia Medical Group in Richmond, Virginia, a group practice with 475 providers—nearly half of them in primary care—has used analytics in conjunction with other health IT solutions in its PHM program. As a result of deploying all of these tools, Bon Secours has seen a 6:1 return on investment, a Phytel case study says.

With the help of a PHM solutions vendor, Bon Secours aggregated data from its clinical information systems and other sources into a population-wide registry that enabled it to implement multiple quality-improvement programs simultaneously. Besides stratifying the population by health risk, the registry allowed care teams to drill down to the data they needed about cohorts and individual patients. This enabled them to monitor their patients' health status and deliver timely, automated interventions.

Bon Secours participates in the MSSP and has value-based contracts with CIGNA and Anthem. These health plans give the organization regular monthly payments for care coordination, and the group has nearly reached the quality threshold necessary for gain sharing with CIGNA. Under its contract with that payer alone, Bon Secours expects to share in annual savings of $4 million, according to Phytel.

Care management

A growing number of group practices have staff members who are dedicated to providing team-based primary care. But these care managers find it difficult to serve all of their high-risk patients. Automated solutions can make the difference between success and failure in this all-important area.

One organization that has made significant progress in automating care management is Northeast Georgia Physicians Group (NGPG). Using a grant from the Center for Medicare and Medicaid Innovation (CMMI),[34] the 200-provider group combined a patient registry and automated messaging with a care-management program for high-risk individuals, a Phytel case study documents.

Focusing first on out-of-control diabetic patients, NGPG assigned a nurse care manager to each one and gave the nurses authority to make certain clinical decisions, such as adjusting medications or dosages. In 120 days, NGPG decreased the HbA1c levels of its nearly 7,000 uncontrolled diabetics by an average of 1.6 points. More than half of the patients achieved significant reductions in A1c levels.

The group used the same automated solutions to engage the patients who visited the ER most frequently. With care managers contacting these patients to determine the reasons for their visits, NGPG was able to decrease their trips to the ER significantly within just three months.

While NGPG didn't measure its ROI directly, it's clear that the ability to prevent diabetic complications and keep people out of the ER can save money for the health-care system. And when payers save money, they will share that with providers under value-based contracts.

Patient engagement

The most potent tool in the population health management tool kit is not a piece of software. It's the patient, whose health behavior often holds the key to his or her future health status. Automation solutions can help care managers reach patients and motivate them to become active participants in their own health care.

The power of patient engagement has been demonstrated by North Mississippi Medical Center, a 650-bed facility in Tupelo, Mississippi, and a winner of the Malcolm Baldrige National Quality Award. In 2012, this organization's ambulatory group, North Mississippi Medical Clinics Inc. (NMMCI), decided to initiate contact with patients prior to office visits and to get them involved in taking better care of themselves between visits, according to Phytel.

NMMCI had an advanced EHR, but that system lacked the population health management tools required to make a difference in patient outcomes. In addition, the patient registry it had been using for years tracked only the patients a physician had seen in the previous thirty days.

After putting a more robust, population-wide registry in place, NMMCI initiated a pilot project aimed at improving the outcomes for seventy-six patients with diabetes who had high HbA1c levels, defined as a value of 9 or greater. The group used analytics with their registry to identify these patients and alert care managers so they could intervene with them prior to office visits.

Once the nurses had their work list, they called the patients and encouraged them to get their lab tests done prior to seeing their providers. The care managers were also able to educate these patients face-to-face after they'd seen their providers. Finally, they sent automated messages to the patients to thank them for their visits and urge them to call back if they had any questions about their plan of care.

The results of this campaign were positive. Of the seventy-six patients who had HbA1c levels > 9.0, thirty-one (41 percent) dropped to below 9. And of the forty-five patients still considered high-risk, thirty-nine received education on how to manage their diabetes more effectively.

Transitions of care

Many hospitals and health-care systems are trying to reduce readmissions to avoid CMS penalties.[35] Hospitals are also paying increased attention to patient satisfaction, which can affect both their reimbursement and their marketing effectiveness. Scores on the Hospital Consumer Assessment of Healthcare Providers and Systems (HCAHPS), the government's twenty-seven-item patient experience survey, are being posted on HospitalCompare, a CMS website for Medicare beneficiaries.[36] And HCAHPS scores are factored into CMS's new value-based purchasing program, which can result in financial bonuses or penalties for hospitals.[37]

Hospitals are also concerned about the patient experience in their emergency departments. When people are satisfied with their ED experience, they're more likely to use the hospital for any procedures or tests they may need in the future. Many hospitals use the Press Ganey patient-satisfaction survey to find out how well their EDs are doing.

Automation tools can be used to boost patient-experience ratings while reducing the likelihood of readmission. One such application sends automated messages to patients within twenty-four hours after discharge from the hospital or ED. The messages ask the patients to complete a short assessment of their experience. They're asked how they're feeling and whether they understand their discharge instructions, have questions about their medications, and have made an appointment to see their primary care doctor. If they have questions, a care manager contacts them later.

Riverside Health System in Newport News, Virginia, has used this system in the ED at Riverside Regional Medical Center (RRMC) since 2012, notes another Phytel case study. In the first year, RRMC raised its ED's overall Press Ganey score from 58 percent to 63 percent and increased its patient recommendation score from 60 percent to 64 percent. At the same time, it improved the quality of care by providing additional support to patients who needed it. Riverside Health System has introduced the solution in the EDs of three other hospitals and plans to launch it in RRMC's inpatient units to boost its HCAHPS scores.

Prevea Health has also applied automation to transitions of care with the help of its two partner hospitals, St. Mary's Hospital Medical Center and St. Vincent's Hospital. Using an automation tool to identify at-risk patients who have just been discharged, Prevea has its care managers contact those patients within twenty-four to seventy-two hours after they leave the hospital. The care managers make sure that the patients understand their medications and their care instructions. This extra attention helps smooth care transitions and prevent readmissions.

How to calculate ROI

Phytel has calculated the ROI that a group of 200 physicians can expect to derive from using its population health management solutions. This ROI comes from a combination of fee-for-service revenue, pay-for-performance incentives, and savings that represent increased revenues under risk contracts. There are also operational savings, but these are redirected into improved care management that supports the other categories of ROI.

In brief, proactive patient outreach uses a population-wide registry and evidence-based clinical protocols to identify care gaps, send automated messages to all patients, and track the results of the contacts.

Quality reporting applies analytics to the registry, allowing users to drill down to individuals and subpopulations and identify opportunities for care improvement. Clinical analytics also makes it easy to gather data and report on quality measures for value-based payment programs.

Care management tools can stratify populations by health risk and identify high-risk patients, and gives care managers tools to execute focused interventions that lower risks and improve outcomes. These tools also allow care managers to view care gaps prior to, during, and after a patient's visit to his or her provider. And enable users to target outreach campaigns to subpopulations that need help, such as diabetic patients who have not received an A1c test in the past six months.

Patient outreach: additional visit revenues

Our hypothetical physician group, divided evenly between primary care doctors and specialists, is caring for about 200,000 active patients. Twenty percent of the population, or 40,000 patients, are covered by insurance contracts that include pay-for-performance (P4P) incentives. Another 15 percent, or 30,000 patients, are covered by risk contracts.

About 45 percent of the fee-for-service population, or 76,500 patients, have not received all recommended care. Automated messaging can successfully contact 80 percent of the patients with care gaps, based on Phytel's experience. Of those people, 20 percent, or 12,240, will make appointments with their provider to receive necessary services, and 15 percent, or 11,475, will return for follow-up visits.

At an average office charge of $85, those visits to fill care gaps generate $2,015,775 in additional revenue for the group. That includes $1,040,400 in revenue from initial visits to help patients adhere to their care plans, and $975,375 from follow-up encounters.

Pay for performance: maximizing incentives

Care management tools drive automated messaging to the entire population, across the gamut from healthy people to those with advanced illnesses. In a P4P population of 40,000 patients, care managers would have to make 247,200 phone calls to reach 80 percent of the patients. At an average 1.5 minutes per call, that task would require 6,180 hours. By not having to make those calls, care managers would be freed to work closely with patients at risk of complications, improving the group's P4P scores.

Let's assume that, by using manual methods of care management, the group was able to qualify for 25 percent of available P4P incentives. At an average rate of $1.50 per member per month (PMPM), the practice would receive just $165,000 of an incentive pool of $660,000 for the year. But if the increased productivity of care managers could help raise that percentage to 95 percent, the group would get $627,000, representing additional P4P revenue of $462,000. If the incentive were raised to $2.00 PMPM in the second year, the extra income would be $616,000; if it rose to $2.50 PMPM, the group would receive an extra $770,000.

Risk contracts: lowering overall costs

As in the P4P example, automated messaging would also give care managers additional time to work with high-risk patients covered by prepaid contracts. Assuming that 30,000 patients were covered under these agreements, 185,400 calls would be required to reach 80 percent of them. At 1.5 minutes per call, the automated messaging would save the nurses 4,635 hours that they could use in care management.

Based on the average costs of care delivery, we calculate that this population would generate medical expenses of about $165 million a year. If a care-management program powered by automation tools could save only 0.5 percent more than could be achieved through manual efforts, that increment would represent a cost decrease of $825,000. Under a financial-risk contract, that additional money drops straight to the group's bottom line.

ROI summary

Looking at the three sources of ROI for our 200-doctor group, we project that the use of PHM automation tools would produce annual revenues of $2,015,775 from fee-for-service visits, $462,000 from P4P, and $825,000 from at-risk contracts. Those amounts add up to $3.3 million, many times the cost of the software for a group of this size.

The staff efficiencies created by automation can also be measured. In the scenario we've described, the group would save 10,815 hours that could otherwise be spent contacting patients. That's equivalent to the annual work of 5.6 full-time care managers. However, no organization would assign nurses to do nothing but dial patients all day long. What happens in groups without automation tools is that most patients simply do not hear from their providers between visits.

The time savings created by automation could result in a hard ROI from lowering the number of care managers. But an organization that is trying to maximize its value-based reimbursement would be wiser to reinvest the time savings in greater productivity for its care managers. By enabling them to intervene with more patients, the organization can achieve ROI by providing more value to payers.

Conclusion

The transition to value-based payment requires a new kind of thinking that equates waste reduction and quality improvement with income. This new attitude must also be applied to thinking about return on investment. The investments that used to produce revenue—and that still do, in many cases—will not necessarily be the ones that will lead to financial success in this new world.

What will generate ROI are investments in information technology that helps organizations work with patients to produce better health outcomes. Care managers are an essential part of this approach, but any population health management initiative that relies on manual methods is doomed to failure. Organizations need electronic tools that automate routine outreach tasks, and they need analytics that automate the process of risk stratification, care-gap identification, and performance measurement. With these tools in hand, they can move forward confidently to claim their share of value-based reimbursement.

The key to creating ROI—and to managing population health—is care coordination, or planned care. The next chapter shows how automation tools can help providers coordinate care for an entire patient population at an affordable cost.

Section 3

Implementing Change

Automating Care Coordination with Health IT

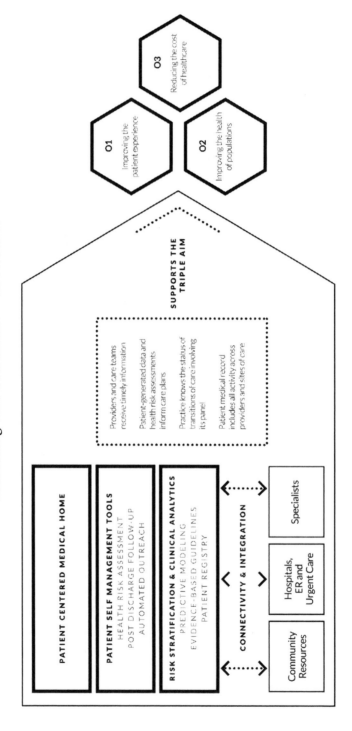

O1
Improving the patient experience

O2
Improving the health of populations

O3
Reducing the cost of healthcare

SUPPORTS THE TRIPLE AIM

Providers and care teams receive timely information

Patient-generated data and health risk assessments inform care plans

Practice knows the status of transitions of care involving its panel

Patient medical record includes all activity across providers and sites of care

PATIENT CENTERED MEDICAL HOME

PATIENT SELF MANAGEMENT TOOLS
HEALTH RISK ASSESSMENT
POST DISCHARGE FOLLOW-UP
AUTOMATED OUTREACH

RISK STRATIFICATION & CLINICAL ANALYTICS
PREDICTIVE MODELING
EVIDENCE-BASED GUIDELINES
PATIENT REGISTRY

CONNECTIVITY & INTEGRATION

Community Resources

Hospitals, ER and Urgent Care

Specialists

Chapter 8

Care Coordination

- *Introduction*: Care coordination, which is vital to both ACOs and patient-centered medical homes (PCMHs), has made progress in US health care—although it can only achieve its full potential through information technology.
- *Defining care coordination*: Care coordination can be defined many different ways. But above all, care coordination is planned care.
- *PGP demonstration*: Medicare's Physician Group Practice demonstration, the precursor of its ACO shared-savings program, provides important lessons on care coordination from leading group practices.
- *Patient-centered medical home*: Designed to rebuild primary care and improve care coordination, the PCMH has proved its value. However, many practices find the approach too expensive without automation. The latest PCMH criteria require a health IT infrastructure that can support the necessary automation tools.
- *Technology use in care coordination*: Current EHRs are often not sufficient for care coordination, and other health IT tools must be deployed, including registries, care-management software, and automated patient-outreach tools.
- *Continuum of care*: For the PCMH to coordinate care across the continuum, the electronic exchange of clinical data is key. Medical homes should use an array of health IT solutions that can help them facilitate care coordination throughout the medical neighborhood.

Despite the recent slowdown in the growth of health costs, the United States still spends far more than other advanced countries do and has less to show for it.[1] Consequently, the government and private payers remain focused on the Triple Aim of reducing the cost of health care, improving population health, and enhancing the patient experience.

The two leading models for transforming health care to achieve these goals are the patient-centered medical home (PCMH) and the accountable care organization (ACO). Care coordination is a fundamental requirement of both approaches,[2] but it has a long way to go before it achieves its potential.

Even within large health-care organizations, care coordination is often poor.[3] In the fragmented medical communities where most care is delivered, coordination among unrelated health-care providers is rudimentary or nonexistent. And while both secure e-mail and patient portals have been around for some time, they are not even beginning to address the coordination of information across health-care entities.

What all of this leads to is tremendous waste, suboptimal outcomes of care, and higher-than-necessary costs. It has been estimated, for example, that 10 percent of direct-care costs could be saved if the patients with the most poorly coordinated care were better managed.[4] On the patient side, they are left frustrated and without the assistance to improve their quality of life.

The challenges of care coordination reflect the fragmentation of the system and the counterproductive financial incentives of health-care providers. Among the main barriers to better coordination are: the tendency of many patients to seek care from multiple providers without having a personal physician engage them as they move across care settings[5]; poor communication between ER physicians and ambulatory-care providers[6]; slow or no communication between inpatient and outpatient providers[7]; inadequate exchange of information between referring doctors and specialists[8]; lack of financial incentives for care coordination[9]; insufficient staff in primary care offices to do care coordination[10]; and suboptimal use of health information technology.[11]

While better use of technology would not be sufficient to overcome all of the obstacles, it is a vital component of care coordination. A study on the development of the patient-centered medical home states:

> Data-driven tools must enable population-based decision-making, facilitate patient tracking, and provide the data to ensure that practices are meeting their clinical goals for patients. Physicians, care coordinators, and their teams must be empowered with tools that allow them to track patients as they interact with other elements of the health care system and to monitor their clinical progress over time.[12]

Another paper on the role of health IT in quality improvement points out:

> Clinical processes must evolve so as to improve care and be more responsive to patients' needs, and HIT's capabilities must evolve along with them. HIT has particular potential in such areas as coordination of care, workflow efficiency and use of teams, clinical decision support, and population health management—all areas offering glimpses of both the potential and the challenges associated with improved HIT use.[13]

This chapter explains what care coordination is and describes some of the lessons that can be derived from health-care organizations that are leaders in building systems of planned care. In addition, we show how the latest information technology is being used to support care coordination.

Defining care coordination

In discussions of care coordination, one may hear it described as the process of guiding patients through the system, of managing the care of patients with chronic diseases, or of trying to help very sick patients stay out of the hospital. Actually, it's all of these things and more. The Agency for Healthcare Research and Quality (AHRQ) offers this definition:

> Care coordination is the deliberate organization of patient care activities between two or more participants (including the patient) involved in a patient's care to facilitate the appropriate delivery of health care services. Organizing care involves the marshaling of personnel and other resources needed to carry out all required patient care activities, and is often managed by the exchange of information among participants responsible for different aspects of care.[14]

The key phrase in this description is "deliberate organization." Whatever its specific application, coordinated care is *planned* care. And "planned" means something that goes beyond a particular doctor's orders or treatment plans. This is planning that may involve multiple providers, care-team members, and of course, the patient.

The components of care coordination, according to AHRQ, include:

- essential care tasks;
- assessment of a patient's care-coordination needs;
- development of a coordinated care plan;
- identification of team members responsible for coordination;
- information exchange across care interfaces;
- interventions that support care coordination;
- monitoring and adjustment of care; and
- evaluation of outcomes, including identification of care-coordination issues.[15]

In addition, AHRQ identifies some key concepts associated with care coordination:

- collaborative relationships among health-care professionals;
- multidisciplinary care teams who contribute specialized knowledge in nonhierarchical relationships;
- continuity of care across clinicians and care settings;

- chronic disease management, which often uses nurse case managers to help patients follow treatment plans and cope with their conditions;
- case management, which depends on a case manager who closely follows high-risk patients; and
- care management, which applies "systems, science, incentives, and information to improve medical practice and help patients manage medical conditions more effectively."

PGP demonstration

To understand how health-care leaders are trying to manage the challenges of care coordination, it is useful to look at the experiences of the ten groups that participated in Medicare's five-year physician group practice (PGP) demonstration.

Officially classified as a pay-for-performance initiative, the PGP pilot turned out to be a precursor of Medicare's shared-savings program for accountable care organizations. Like ACOs, the PGPs were eligible to split savings with Medicare if they met certain quality benchmarks and the savings exceeded 2 percent of expected costs. In the demonstration project, participants could keep up to 80 percent of the savings they generated, depending on how well they did in meeting the program's quality goals.[16]

In the final year of the five-year demonstration, seven of the ten groups achieved benchmark performance on all of the thirty-two quality goals. The other three groups passed the threshold on at least thirty goals. That year, four of the PGPs generated Medicare savings of $36.2 million in total, and earned performance payments of $29.4 million.[17] Over the five-year period, the participating practices saved a combined $137.8 million and received $107.6 million from Medicare.[18]

The PGPs attributed their savings to a number of factors, including organizational structure, investments in care management and care redesign, more intensive diagnostic coding, and changes in market conditions.[19]

Each of the PGPs that achieved savings used different care-management strategies. For example, the Dartmouth-Hitchcock Clinic in Lebanon, New Hampshire, focused on evidence-based care initiatives, including better use of care alerts, changing work flow for support staff, and using nurse case managers to work with high-risk patients. St. John's Clinic in Springfield, Missouri, used a comprehensive patient registry, care alerts at the point of care, a case manager in the emergency department to plan transitions of care, and a care team dedicated to patients with congestive heart failure.[20]

Marshfield Clinic

The Marshfield Clinic, a 730-doctor clinic in Marshfield, Wisconsin, generated about half of the total savings in the PGP demonstration. The group has been using an electronic health record since 1985 and has long-running quality improvement programs.

For the demonstration project, Marshfield focused on reducing hospital admissions, partly by expanding its telephonic case-management program for patients who had heart failure and hypertension complications. Also, the clinic expanded its anticoagulation drug therapy management program, designed to reduce costly complications of warfarin therapy. Marshfield introduced partial open-access scheduling and redesigned care processes for chronic disease patients to ensure they received all recommended care.

Electronic tools of various kinds are essential to population health management at Marshfield. For example, the clinic's EHR automatically generates an intervention list for each physician that identifies high-risk patients with multiple chronic conditions. Marshfield also uses electronic prescribing, a data warehouse, analytics, patient registries, and care-management software.[21]

During its first year of participating in the demonstration, Marshfield reduced hospitalizations of patients in the anticoagulation-management program by 29 percent. Satisfaction among patients enrolled in care-management programs exceeded 85 percent.[22]

Geisinger Clinic

Another participant in the pilot, the Geisinger Clinic in Danville, Pennsylvania, is part of a health system that includes the 367-bed Geisinger Medical Center and two other hospitals. The Geisinger Clinic employs about 640 physicians in forty-one practice sites.

Geisinger already had disease-management programs in place when it joined the PGP demonstration. The group wanted to expand those programs and extend them to Medicare patients. Among the conditions its programs addressed were asthma, chronic kidney disease, chronic obstructive pulmonary disease, heart failure, diabetes, hypertension, osteoporosis, and smoking cessation. Additionally, Geisinger introduced a case-management program for high-risk, complex patients.[23]

In the PGP pilot, Geisinger sought to reduce hospital admissions and readmissions through disease and case management, enhanced use of its EHR, and an advanced medical home model known as ProvenHealth Navigator. Specifically, Geisinger emphasized patient-centered, team-based care across the continuum, transitions of care coordination, readmission risk screening, and telephonic care management and device-based remote monitoring for heart failure patients. It also redesigned its systems of care to reflect evidence-based guidelines.[24]

Technology is central to Geisinger's approach. For example, the group utilizes patient registries in conjunction with its EHR to identify and resolve patients' care gaps. These registries are used to initiate interventions such as letters, referrals, laboratory test orders, and secure e-mails to ensure that patients receive needed preventive and chronic care. The alerting of patients about pneumococcal and influenza immunizations has been particularly successful.

The Geisinger EHR also provides best-practice alerts to providers at the point of care. Physicians can view a summary of the patient's care, and they receive reminders about needed tests and other interventions. Equally important, they're in close touch with the care managers who are handling their most difficult cases.

Lessons learned

Geisinger's and Marshfield's successes in the Medicare pilot depended largely on their well-executed coordinated-care approaches and their effective use of information technology. Geisinger had two advantages over Marshfield: it owned hospitals, which made it easier to coordinate care across the inpatient/outpatient boundary, and it owned a health plan, which provided an incentive to lower costs for plan members.

RTI International, the company that analyzed the PGP pilot for the Centers for Medicare and Medicaid Services (CMS), drew a few other lessons from the test[25]:

- Medicare patients often have several comorbidities that need to be treated simultaneously. Therefore, group practices must address the need for complex care management that goes beyond traditional disease management for single conditions.
- Complex care management could be enhanced by combining disease-specific patient registries, or by using registries that encompass all patients.
- Planned visits can be facilitated through the use of data systems (e.g., registries and electronic health records) that analyze data and provide physicians and other clinicians with pertinent information about the patient prior to a visit. A visit-planner report may, for example, provide a list of overdue tests for a patient that could be performed prior to a visit.

- Key change opportunities include increasing patient engagement, expanding care management, improving care transitions, and expanding the role of nonphysician providers.

Patient-centered medical home

The patient-centered medical home (PCMH), an approach designed to rebuild primary care and improve care coordination, has become a major focus of health-care reform. The National Committee for Quality Assurance (NCQA) has provided PCMH recognition to more than 29,500 clinicians in 6,037 practice sites, and more practices continue to apply for recognition.[26]

The Centers for Medicare and Medicaid Services (CMS) is also encouraging the spread of the PCMH approach. In 2011, CMS launched an advanced primary care practice demonstration that includes private payers and that pays care-coordination fees to physicians. By the end of the three-year pilot, 1,200 practices serving over 900,000 Medicare beneficiaries are expected to be participating.[27] Meanwhile, Blue Cross and Blue Shield plans support PCMH in forty states, and more than 5 million Blues members have medical homes.[28]

A published analysis of seven PCMH pilots showed that they all achieved cost savings, quality improvements, or both. For example, hospitalization rates were reduced by 6 to 19 percent, ER visits decreased by up to 29 percent, and cost savings ranged from $71 to $640 per patient.[29]

More recently, the Patient-Centered Primary Care Collaborative (PCPCC) posted data indicating that medical homes improve quality and lower costs. For example:

- Blue Cross Blue Shield of Michigan found that practices with full PCMH implementation had savings of $26.37 per member per month.
- In the Military Health System, the PCMH model led to 6.8 percent fewer ED visits, a 13 percent reduction in pharmacy costs, and a 16 percent decrease in ancillary costs.

- At UPMC Health Plan in Pennsylvania, a PCMH pilot was associated with 5.1 percent fewer ED visits, a smaller increase in hospitalizations than non-PCMH practices, 12.5 percent fewer readmissions, and a 160 percent return on investment.
- CareFirst BlueCross Blue Shield of Maryland saved $98 million on its PCMH initiative.[30]

Role of care coordination

Coordinated, planned care is a key feature of medical homes. According to a PCPCC report, "In studies of the medical home, care coordination has emerged as one of the key pillars of programs that have demonstrated improved outcomes and lowered costs."[31]

But unless a medical home is part of a large group or a health-care system, it typically encounters difficulties in paying for care coordinators. Today's fee-for-service health-care system does not compensate providers for most activities outside of face-to-face encounters with clinicians.

According to one study, the annual cost of care coordination in a pediatric practice is $6,600 for each full-time-equivalent primary care provider. The duties of a care manager in such a practice would include:

- identifying the short- and long-term needs of each child,
- developing a written care plan and working with the family to determine action steps,
- implementing the care plan with the family and coordinating with other providers,
- ensuring continuity of care, and
- evaluating the care plan to identify new needs and strategies.[32]

Some care-coordination costs are related to work flow. For example, Greenhouse Internal Medicine, a five-physician practice in Philadelphia that participated in a medical home pilot, hired a nurse educator to help patients manage their chronic conditions. The educator used the medical assistants in the practice to reach as many patients as possible. The project ran into difficulties, partly because of the complexity of changing work flow and also because data from the patients' action plans had to be entered manually into the group's EHR. The practice spent $7,500 to create a special electronic form for this purpose.

Greenhouse's doctors felt the self-management project was helping some patients, but less than 30 percent of the diabetic patients who visited the office set self-management goals, and few people entered home measurements of blood pressure or glucose levels on the practice website, as requested. Moreover, the practice's investment in care coordination would not have been possible without the extra reimbursement it received for being in the medical-home pilot.[33]

Insurance companies have been willing to foot the bill in pilots, and some are paying doctors extra for providing medical homes. Governmental entities are also encouraging the model. Besides the already-cited Medicare demonstration, the North Carolina Medicaid program pays a community organization to provide care managers to primary care physicians, who also receive care-coordination fees.[34] Similarly, the Vermont Blueprint for Health uses community health teams to supplement the efforts of its medical homes.[35]

Without this kind of external support, however, it's too expensive for most practices to hire the requisite number of extra support staff. According to one estimate, the average PCMH requires 4.25 full-time-equivalent staff members per FTE provider, compared to 2.68 staff per provider in a typical primary care practice.[36]

Technology solutions

One way to meet this challenge is to use information technology wherever possible to automate care coordination and care management. For example, University of North Carolina (UNC) Health Care, a large multispecialty practice, has received NCQA recognition as a level 3 medical home. The group uses an EHR, a patient registry, a patient-health survey, and care-management software to improve the health of its population.[37]

UNC's care-management application (called "Visit Planner") provides care-team members with automated prompts to assess patient needs. It also coordinates and identifies team-member roles throughout a patient visit.

Groups that have automated some care-management functions, such as patient outreach, have obtained a return on investment by generating additional visits for needed chronic and preventive care. As a result, one study indicates, patients are more likely to receive recommended care.

Using data from Prevea Health, a large multispecialty group, in Green Bay, Wisconsin, researchers found that patients who received automated telephone messages were more likely to have both a chronic-care office visit and an appropriate test than patients who were not contacted. Compared to a control group of noncontacted patients, about three times as many diabetic patients who were successfully contacted had both a visit and an HbA1c test. And twice as many patients with hypertension who received this intervention had both a visit and a systolic blood pressure reading recorded in Prevea's EHR.[38]

Another benefit of automating care management is that it eliminates much of the routine work, giving care managers and care coordinators time to provide services to more of the patients who need their help. While this doesn't reduce the cost of labor, it can increase a practice's value-based reimbursement by raising quality scores and preventing complications that generate higher health costs.

New NCQA criteria

The health IT infrastructure required for this kind of automation is imbedded in NCQA's 2014 PCMH recognition criteria. Among other things, these guidelines require the use of health IT in care coordination and care transitions, as follows:

Test tracking and follow-up: Providers must record lab and radiology orders in the EHR and incorporate the majority of lab results in structured data fields. NCQA also requires applicants to track lab and imaging tests from the time they're ordered until results are available. One method is to flag orders not accompanied by results in the EHR.

Referral tracking and follow-up: Providers must send an electronic summary of care record to other providers in more than 50 percent of referrals. The referring doctor must also give the consultant or specialist a range of information, including lab results and the current care plan, that can be transferred from the electronic record. A critical factor is the ability to track referrals until the consultant's report is available—a difficult objective to achieve without the use of an EHR.

Coordinating care transitions: Providers must exchange key clinical information electronically with other care providers, including hospitals, ERs, extended care facilities, and nursing homes. Providers must have the ability to identify patients with unplanned hospital admissions and emergency-department visits, to share clinical information with admitting hospitals and EDs, and to consistently obtain patient-discharge summaries from the hospital and other facilities.[39]

Additionally, the NCQA guidelines require patients to have electronic access to their health records and include criteria related to team-based care and population health management that would be impossible to meet without health IT tools. For example, care teams must support all patients in self-management, self-efficacy, and behavior change and must identify which patients need interventions from care managers.

Technology use in care coordination

As health-care organizations form ACOs and medical homes, they have to coordinate care effectively across populations and care settings. A consensus report on combining these two care-delivery models observes that care coordination will be the linchpin of health-care transformation:

The effective coordination of a patient's health care services is a key component of high-quality, efficient care. It provides value to patients, professionals and the health care system by improving the quality, appropriateness, timeliness and efficiency of decision-making and care activities, thereby affecting the experience, quality and cost of health care.[40]

The consensus report also emphasizes the role of health IT in care coordination, while asserting that the current EHR is insufficient for this purpose.

Anchoring the electronic health record (EHR) in the traditional visit-based care delivery model limits the potential of the medical home to generate paradigm-shifting care delivery transformation and the positive outcomes it promises ... Health IT requires new functional capabilities, such as multiple team member access and permissions, care management workflow support, integrated personal health records, registry functionalities, clinical decision support, measurement of quality and efficiency, and robust reporting.[41]

The bulk of the technologies required to achieve these goals are already available. Among the reasons they're not being properly deployed in most cases are these:

- Electronic health records are not designed to do population health management or care coordination.
- Registries tend to be focused on patients with particular conditions, rather than entire populations.
- Care-management work-flow support is still a relatively new concept, but one that more and more groups are embracing.

Key building blocks

As noted earlier, various forms of information technology, including registries, care-management software, and automated patient-outreach tools have all been deployed successfully, in conjunction with EHRs, to manage patient populations.

The automated stratification of patients into health-risk categories is especially important to groups seeking to do population health management. For example, UNC Healthcare uses a health risk assessment (HRA) survey to find out how sick each of its patients with diabetes is. Then it uses an advanced patient registry and evidence-based algorithms to drive team-based care for each of those patients, depending on the severity of his or her condition.[42]

Many practices use electronic registries to supplement their EHRs. These registries compile lists of subpopulations that need particular kinds of preventive and chronic care, such as annual mammograms for women over 40 or HbA1c tests at particular intervals for diabetic patients. The continuously updated data in the registries come from EHRs, practice-management systems, or a combination of the two. Evidence-based clinical protocols, which can be customized by physician practices, trigger alerts in the registries. When a registry is linked to an outbound messaging system, patients are notified by automated telephone, e-mail, or text messages to contact their physician for an appointment. Some registries can also send actionable data to care teams prior to patient visits.[43]

The use of technology to automate patient education and to prompt certain actions can improve compliance, health behavior, and self-management of chronic diseases. A 2007 AHRQ report on the use of information technology in primary care noted:

> An example of automation to support better individual patient care would be the automatic generation of patient education handouts (including and utilizing patient-specific data and information). Once an action is

145

determined to be appropriate for better care, the health IT system should produce the action based on patient data, in many cases without even requiring provider interaction. An example would be the production of a mailing list for all diabetic patients who have not had an eye exam in the last year.[44]

One group practice that has been especially successful in using technology to automate population health management is Northeast Georgia Physicians Group (NGPG), the largest multispecialty practice in its region. As part of an initiative to have all of its primary care sites recognized as patient-centered medical homes, NGPG in 2012 adopted several automation tools to scale up care coordination and care management to its entire population. These included an application that combined a registry and care-gap identification with automated messaging to alert patients who needed to be seen for preventive or chronic care. In addition, NGPG used a reporting tool that not only measured organizational performance but also allowed care managers to spot patients who needed help in managing their chronic conditions. Another automation program gave the care managers additional tools to risk-stratify patients and to develop personalized care interventions for those who required them.[45]

The initial results were promising. In the six months between January and July 2013, NPGP tested the outreach and care-management applications in ten sites. The care managers used them on a daily basis to track and target 860 diabetic patients who had an HbA1c > 9. By the end of the study period, NGPG had helped 412 of those patients lower that value to less than 9 percent. Including all participants, the patients' A1c values declined by an average of 1.3 percentage points.

Orlando Health, a major health-care system in Orlando, Florida, has deployed the same set of applications that NGPG uses to improve population health management in a clinically integrated network of physicians. Having recognized that the network's multiple EHRs were inadequate for the task, Orlando Health combined them with automation tools for patient outreach, reporting, and care management.

Before acquiring these tools, the health-care system was challenged by the NCQA requirements for gaining recognition of its primary care sites as patient-centered medical homes. It was very time-consuming to create custom reports for care management manually, and the data were often incomplete and out-of-date. By being able to generate reports from a registry in near-real time themselves, the care managers gained an indispensable tool for targeting the patients who needed their help most. Automated messaging to subgroups of patients with care gaps also reduced the care managers' routine tasks, allowing them to spend more time with patients. These tools enabled Orlando Health to scale up its population health management efforts without adding care managers to the fifteen it already had.[46]

The overall lesson to be drawn from the efforts to improve care coordination is that it's difficult to get very far without the use of information technology. The identification of patients with particular conditions, health risk assessments, the ability to send care-gap alerts to providers, the care management of chronically ill patients, tailored patient education, and persistent reminders to patients to get the care they need—all of these interventions require some degree of automation to be performed in a timely, consistent, cost-effective manner.

Continuum of care

The PCPCC views the patient-centered medical home as the hub of the "medical neighborhood." That ecosystem includes both health-care providers (e.g., primary care doctors, specialists, behavioral health providers, hospitals, home health agencies, and long-term-care facilities) and community organizations that encourage healthy living, wellness, and safe environments (e.g., YMCAs, schools, faith-based organizations, employers, and public health agencies).[47]

For primary care practices to coordinate care and manage population health effectively within this medical neighborhood, they must have a health IT infrastructure, the PCPCC notes. The key HIT tools required for this approach include EHRs, patient registries, health information exchanges (HIEs), tools for risk stratification, automated outreach and referral tracking, patient portals, telehealth applications, and remote patient monitoring systems.

HIEs can facilitate care coordination where they are available. In addition, an increasing number of organizations are starting to exchange clinical summaries via the Direct secure messaging protocol.

New automation tools can help providers improve transitions of care and track referrals across the medical neighborhood. For example, some organizations use an application that messages patients shortly after a hospital discharge. The patients are asked if they have questions about their discharge instructions or medications. This tool can be used to automatically transfer patients to a care-team member or can trigger outbound calls from their physician or primary care practice. Riverside Health System in Newport News, Virginia, is one of the health-care systems that have made effective use of this solution to raise its patient-satisfaction scores.

Medicare to Reward Physicians for Care Coordination

To counter the financial disincentives for care coordination, the Centers for Medicare and Medicaid Services (CMS) has announced that, starting in January 2015, it will begin paying physicians to coordinate care for patients who have two or more chronic conditions and are in the Medicare fee-for-service program.[48] One-third of Medicare beneficiaries have two or more chronic diseases, and 70% of Medicare patients are in the fee for service program.[49]

In return for a care coordination fee of about $42 per patient per month, physicians will be expected to assess patients' medical, psychological and social needs; check whether they are taking medications as prescribed; monitor the care provided by other doctors; and ensure smooth transitions of care when patients move from a hospital to their home or a nursing home.

Patients can decide whether they want to have their care coordinated. Those who do will pay 20% of the fee for those services.

Conclusion

The interventions explored in this chapter are all necessary but not sufficient to attain the goals of the Triple Aim: improve the experience of care, improve the health of populations, and reduce the per capita costs of care.[50] US health care is still in the early stages of organizing itself so that, for example, providers communicate easily with each other about patient care across care settings and between organizations. Patients are also just beginning to gain access to their own medical records and communicate online with their physicians.[51]

Nevertheless, the recent advances in health IT and further developments in this vital field will continue to support and enhance care coordination as it expands across the spectrum of care. Assuming that payment methods also change to support coordinated care, we can look forward to a proliferation of new IT tools that will help turn the vision of affordable, high-quality health care for all into a reality.

Another key component of health-care transformation that is just starting to be applied in a rigorous way is the Lean approach to process improvement. The next chapter shows how some organizations are starting to use Lean thinking and IT-driven automation to improve care management.

Stratifying Populations to Achieve Lean Care Management

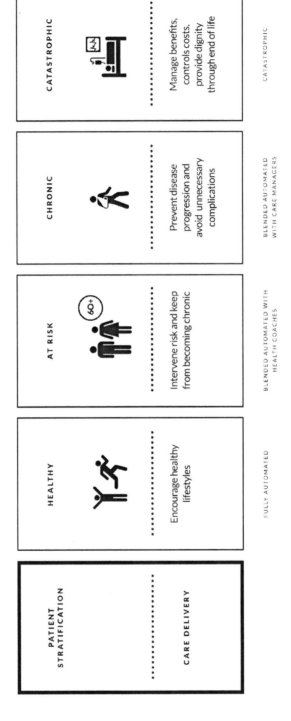

	HEALTHY	AT RISK	CHRONIC	CATASTROPHIC
PATIENT STRATIFICATION				
CARE DELIVERY	Encourage healthy lifestyles	Intervene risk and keep from becoming chronic	Prevent disease progression and avoid unnecessary complications	Manage benefits, controls costs, provide dignity through end of life
	FULLY AUTOMATED	BLENDED AUTOMATED WITH HEALTH COACHES	BLENDED AUTOMATED WITH CARE MANAGERS	CATASTROPHIC

Chapter 9

Lean Care Management

- *Introduction:* Care teams have been shown to help high-performing practices raise their capacity and productivity, while improving quality and care coordination. The Lean approach to continuous quality improvement, coupled with IT-driven automation, may provide the missing ingredients to make the care-team model an economic winner.
- *A Lean foundation in health care:* The key concepts of Lean thinking—including value-stream mapping, continuous flow, and continuous improvement—can be applied to health care. The Lean care-management approach is now starting to gain traction among leading-edge groups.
- *High-performing practices:* These practices exhibit many elements of the Lean approach, including the reduction of non-value-added work steps, the "voice of the customer (patient)," and rapid experiments with solutions to improve processes. Using Lean techniques, these practices have figured out how to allow team members to utilize the full range of their abilities and skills.
- *Lean care management:* There is no one-size-fits-all approach that will work for every group. But pre-visit planning and care coordination, along with work-flow mapping and reengineering, help some practices increase efficiency and reduce waste.
- *Automation in Lean processes:* Incorporating health IT into Lean processes can enable care teams to manage entire populations. Automation tools for risk stratification, patient outreach, and care

management can leverage the capabilities of care managers and enable physicians and all care-team members to work at the top of their licenses.

Primary care practices must be reengineered to achieve the Triple Aim of improving the experience of care, improving population health, and reducing the cost of care. As new value-based payment and delivery models continue to expand, practices have strong incentives to take on the necessary reengineering. In addition, shortages of generalist physicians in many areas of the country, coupled with increasing patient demand, offer additional pressure to redesign the current fee-for-service primary care model.

One promising alternative to the traditional model involves the use of care teams that include a variety of clinical and nonclinical staff members. By sharing responsibility for care among team members, high-performing practices have been able to increase their capacity and productivity. There's also a growing body of evidence that this model can improve quality and care coordination.[1]

Launching the team care model can be culturally and financially challenging as health-care organizations traverse the path from volume-based payment (e.g., fee-for-service) to value-based payment (e.g., population-based quality performance and cost savings). Effective care coordination can require additional staff and technology that few small practices can afford.[2] Strategic leaders recognize that investing in team-based care today is imperative for success tomorrow as value-based payment becomes more dominant.

Practices managing population health typically need additional RNs to serve as care managers for patients with complex chronic diseases. In addition, family medicine societies and the National Committee for Quality Assurance (NCQA) recently recommended that behavioral health specialists be integrated into the patient-centered medical home (PCMH), an increasingly prevalent model that emphasizes team-based care.[3] And it's not unusual for high-performing practices to include pharmacists, nutritionists, diabetes educators, health coaches, and social workers.[4]

Not all of these kinds of professionals are included on all care teams. Nevertheless, based on the literature and interviews with practice administrators, researchers have calculated that a PCMH care team has an average staffing ratio of 4.25 staff per full-time primary care physician. By comparison, the staffing ratio in the typical primary care practice is 2.68:1.[5]

Some health plans pay care-coordination fees or incentivize practices that have been recognized as a PCMH.[6] Value-based reimbursement may also be available in the form of shared-savings and risk contracts with a quality component.[7] To the extent that primary care practices can deliver that kind of value, while also increasing their own efficiency, they should do well in the emerging world of value-based reimbursement. In many cases, that should justify the extra overhead that fully capable care teams add to practices.

Today most practices are using manual methods of care management that don't achieve the labor-saving potential of health IT. And unless they have a systematic approach to process improvement, they're often not as efficient as they could be in engaging everyone in their patient panels

To maximize efficiency and achieve the Triple Aim, primary care providers should consider two emerging trends: *IT-driven automation* and *continuous quality improvement* based on Lean and Six Sigma principles. These approaches, while common in other industries, have only recently begun to gain traction in health care. And they are already showing promise as health-care organizations transition from the model of the physician who has sole responsibility for providing care to the care-team model, in which many health-care tasks are delegated to nonphysicians.

Lean thinking goes back decades to the Toyota production model. Later associated with Six Sigma, which focuses on reducing defects and variations in processes, Lean is a continuous quality improvement method that relies on motivating frontline workers to reduce cycle time through waste elimination. A growing number of health-care organizations have fully adopted Lean principles to improve quality and reduce waste by reengineering work flows, and many other providers are getting started.

Automation is not required to apply Lean in health care. But automation tools and other types of health IT can be powerful adjuncts to the transformation of health care based on the Lean approach. Health IT solutions can be used to automate many routine tasks of care management, increasing the productivity of care teams.

For example, it's inefficient for a health-care organization to have care managers call every patient with gaps in recommended care. Automated phone, texting, or e-mail messaging could reach the vast majority of these patients, significantly reducing the amount of staff time that must be devoted to this task. As a result, the organization could employ fewer care managers or could deploy its existing ones more effectively to help high-risk patients.

The combination of Lean with automation can boost care teams' productivity and can eliminate much of the waste in health care. This chapter explains the basic tenets of this approach.

A Lean foundation in health care

The Toyota production system, which began in the 1950s, was originally called "just-in-time production" and was later rebranded as Lean. After Toyota used this manufacturing approach to catch up to and later surpass the US automakers, many other companies began to emulate its methods.[8]

The key concepts of Lean thinking include:

- *Value:* Define value from the customer's perspective. Products should be designed for and with customers, should suit the purpose, and be set at the right price.
- *Value stream:* Each step in production must produce "value" for the customer, eliminating all sources of waste.
- *Flow:* The system must flow continuously and without interruption. Flow depends on materials being delivered, as and when they are needed, to the quality required.

- *Pull:* The process must be flexible, producing what customers need when they need it.
- *Perfection:* The aim is perfection. Lean thinking creates an environment of continuous improvement, emphasizing suggestions from workers and learning from previous mistakes.[9]

Several Lean principles are applicable to health care. First, work flow is analyzed and broken down into a series of steps so that any failure in the process can be easily identified. Second, problems are addressed immediately through rapid experimentation with proposed solutions. Third, the ideas that succeed are spread throughout the organization. Fourth and most important, people at all levels of the organization are expected to contribute suggestions for improvement and to participate in testing these "countermeasures" to solve problems.[10]

Gaining the cooperation of frontline staff is not easy or natural in many organizations, especially in health care. Health care is organized along hierarchical lines that can be difficult to break down. In both physician practices and hospitals, physicians stand at the top of the clinical pyramid, with all other clinical staff deferring to them. Nonclinical staff report to administrators and practice managers and also defer to physicians in doctor-owned practices.

Lean thinking requires that these hierarchies be flattened for the purposes of quality improvement. Management must give employees the freedom to critique existing processes and to suggest ways to improve them. Physicians, too, must be willing to delegate tasks to care teams and to let them find ways to improve the work flow and add value to the process.

Even without the addition of Lean, physicians may find it hard to accept the idea of delegating some of their duties to care teams in patient-centered medical homes. In a paper evaluating the national medical home demonstration project of the American Academy of Family Physicians (AAFP), the authors noted:

> We found that changing roles was perhaps most difficult
> for physicians, who believed deeply that primary care
> doctoring was based on a strong, trusting relationship
> between a patient and a physician. Sharing that relationship
> with other practice staff members was, for many, a
> significant challenge to their identity as physicians.[11]

There are other cultural changes that practices must make as they transition
from a physician-dominated model to a care-team model. In an appendix
to the study cited above, the researchers note that the leaders of one practice
in the demonstration project ran into challenges when they tried to use
their registry in population health management, "largely due to difficulty
in reassigning roles and responsibilities to the existing mix of staff."[12]

Engaging frontline employees to be involved in process improvement
poses another cultural challenge, but when leadership is persistent, the
effort pays off: the Illinois-based Christie Clinic, for example, worked on
incorporating Lean concepts for several years before its efforts bore fruit.
The organization has divided its 800 employees, including 160 providers,
into seventy-one site-based teams that work on process improvement. In a
two-year period, these teams made 2,000 improvement suggestions, and
most of those have been implemented.[13]

In a research paper from the Institute for Health Technology Transformation,
Christie Clinic CEO Alan Gleghorn said that the key to applying Lean
in his organization was to create an environment where it was safe for
frontline employees to propose process improvements. They also had to
be told that this was expected of them as part of their jobs, he added.[14]

Lean gains traction in health care

The first big application of Lean principles to ambulatory care occurred
around 2000. That was when the Boston-based Institute for Healthcare
Improvement (IHI) launched a three-year initiative to redesign primary
care at forty practice sites across the country. The program aimed to

remove barriers to patient access, reduce waste and inefficiency, and improve patient-doctor communications, among other goals. Open-access scheduling, team care, non-visit care via phone and e-mail, and practice "huddles" to plan daily work were all part of the game plan.[15]

Clinical staff received new roles and enhanced responsibilities, and the care-team approach necessitated the addition of staff in many practices. But doctors had more time to spend with patients, the patients were happier, and the practices ran more smoothly.

Many aspects of the IHI program were later incorporated into the PCMH approach, which got off the ground in 2006, when the AAFP started its demonstration project. Meanwhile, a number of health-care organizations were already experimenting with Lean thinking. The better-known health-care systems that have tried Lean to date include Thedacare, Virginia Mason Medical Center, Group Health Cooperative, and Cleveland Clinic.[16]

ThedaCare, a Wisconsin organization that also participated in the IHI project, has founded the ThedaCare Center for Healthcare Value (TCHV), which disseminates its knowledge of Lean and brings together members of TCHV's Healthcare Value Network to exchange insights. In the past two years, the Healthcare Value Network has grown from fourteen to sixty member organizations.[17]

High-performing practices

Several recent studies of high-performing primary care practices have examined the characteristics that enable them to deliver high-quality care efficiently. While none of these studies looks at these practices through the lens of Lean principles, many of them have absorbed Lean thinking into their approach. Other practices—notably, those that have studied the Virginia Mason and ThedaCare models—are consciously imbedding Lean into process improvement.

The high-performing practices discussed in these studies all use care teams. Those teams not only improve care delivery but also provide the environment required for the implementation of Lean processes. So before we examine how the Lean approach can be applied to care management, we'll take a look at how care teams transform primary care.

Performing at top of license

The care-team approach requires that practices think about how best to use each team member to provide better care with less waste. A cardinal principle is to enable care-team members to work at the top level of their training, experience, and ability. For example, physicians should not be doing clerical work that does not require their level of knowledge. Nurses should be empowered to do as much as possible within the limits of their licensure. And lower-level employees can also be trained to perform important functions for the care team.

A study funded by the Robert Wood Johnson Foundation, for example, found that many high-performing groups train medical assistants (MAs) to do pre-visit chart reviews, identify patients with gaps in care, and contact them via calls or letters. Some MAs who received extra training also act as health coaches for patients with chronic conditions. And MAs in some groups lead daily "huddles" of care teams to plan the day's activities. Using MAs for these kinds of tasks has been shown to improve rates of preventive services and outcomes of care.

RNs in these practices provide intensive support for high-risk patients with chronic diseases, follow up on patients discharged from the hospital, and coordinate complex specialty care. They also work with patients who have multiple conditions and medications.

In this model, physicians, physician assistants, and nurse practitioners can perform their indispensable diagnostic and treatment functions, while other team members prepare patients for their visits and help them with their care plans afterward.[18]

Another study finds that the common characteristics of high-performing practices are proactive planned care, shared clerical tasks, improved communication, and improved team functioning.

The twenty-three study sites built their capacity to serve patients by giving nurses and other nonphysician clinicians partial responsibility for delivering care. For example, at North Shore Physicians Group (NSPG) in the Boston area, MAs perform an expanded range of functions during the rooming process. These include medication review, agenda setting, form completion, and closing care gaps. MAs review health-monitoring reminders, give immunizations, and book appointments for mammograms and DXA scans for osteoporosis.

Clinica Family Health Services, based in Lafayette, Colorado, has created standing orders so RNs can diagnose and treat simple problems such as strep infections, ear infections, and urinary-tract infections on their own. Nonprofessional health coaches provide patient education and counseling to help patients with chronic conditions set goals and formulate action plans.[19]

Care-coordinator model

Another study analyzes three different approaches to team-based care in primary care practices. The first is the "top-of-license model" described earlier. The second is an "enhanced traditional model," in which nurses, MAs, and front-office staff are organized to support the physician in nontraditional ways. The third is a "care-coordinator model," which is designed for population health management.

In the latter approach, the care team includes a care coordinator, usually a nurse, who works for multiple providers. The care coordinator's main tasks are to coordinate patient transitions in care and to manage high-risk patients. The coordinator also coaches patients who manage their own conditions poorly.

The nurses on the care team perform a number of high-level functions, including identifying care gaps, administering EKGs and immunizations, doing cognitive and mobility assessments, and supporting patients between visits.

This care-coordination approach helped increase one practice's mammography screening rates from 37 percent to 70 percent and the blood pressure control of its diabetic patients from 39 percent to 72 percent over a three-year period. But the practice had to reduce the number and role of care coordinators because of financial difficulty in supporting the model with no extra reimbursement from payers.[20]

Automation in Practice

The use of automation has helped a number of health-care organizations improve their care-management processes and achieve better patient outcomes. While it's still rare for clinics to combine automation with Lean principles of continuous quality improvement, early evidence indicates that this would be an even more effective method to increase efficiency and cut waste than automation alone.

Here are a few examples of how organizations have used automation tools to improve their ability to manage population health.

North Mississippi Medical Clinics (NMMCI), a branch of North Mississippi Medical Center in Tupelo, Mississippi, operates a regional network of thirty-eight primary and specialty-care clinics. To improve its care management, NMMCI purchased a patient registry and automation applications that it interfaced with its EHR, according to a Phytel case study.

Care managers used the registry to identify patients who had poorly controlled diabetes. An automation tool generated work lists showing all preventive services and lab tests required for patients in that category who were scheduled to visit in the next two days. The care managers communicated via e-mail and messaged the patients and encouraged them to get any necessary lab work done before their visit. Work flows were automated and standardized so that no patients slipped between the cracks.

As a result of this campaign, thirty-one of the seventy-six patients who originally had HbA1c levels > 9 are now below that level. Most of the other at-risk patients have received specific education on how to manage their diabetes more effectively.

Prevea Health, a 180-doctor multispecialty group in Green Bay, Wisconsin, needed a way to reach out to chronic-disease patients who had care gaps but did not make appointments to see their providers. Care-management processes were largely manual, making it very difficult to engage all of these patients on a regular basis.

Prevea acquired a population health management solution that included a registry and related technology. Through an interface, the group's EHR populated the registry automatically with demographic and clinical information. Using embedded clinical protocols, a program linked to the registry triggered automated messaging to patients who had care gaps in the areas of diabetes and hypertension. Those patients who were contacted made office appointments at two to three times the rate of noncontacted patients.

The key lesson of Prevea's experience is that the ability to identify patients with care gaps must be coupled with automated outreach capabilities to improve compliance.[21]

Bon Secours Virginia Medical Group (BSVMG), a hospital-owned multispecialty group with more than one hundred locations in and around Richmond, Virginia, has used a care-team approach and the patient-centered medical home model to prepare for value-based reimbursement, a Phytel case study notes.

BSVMG uses an outside registry connected to its EHR for risk stratification and other applications for identifying patient-care gaps. In addition, its population health management solution suggests appropriate interventions for subpopulations of patients. Because these interventions can be automated, care teams are able to communicate with many patients at once and to implement multiple quality improvement programs simultaneously. An analytic application is also being deployed to measure the performance of providers, sites, and the entire practice.

Partly as a result of the process improvements enabled by automation, BSVMG has been able to succeed in its performance-based contracts with commercial payers. Under a contract with just one health plan, the group expects to generate annual savings of $4 million that it will share in. Meanwhile, the increased visits by patients with care gaps have generated more than $7 million in incremental revenue.

Overall, the experience of these and other groups has shown that automation tools can increase the effectiveness and efficiency of care management. In addition, the automation of work flows guarantees that organizations will be able to reach most of the targeted patients who need preventive, chronic care, or other services.

Lean care management

There is no one-size-fits-all method on how to create an optimal care team or design the work flows that enable the team to deliver the best care with maximal efficiency. Practices vary by specialty, size, resources, payer mix, and the composition of their patient population. The use of information technology and automation can vary dramatically from one practice to another. And the medical neighborhoods in which practices operate—including whether or not they're part of a health-care system— also influence the way care teams function.[22]

All of this only begins to explain the nuances that must be considered when one sets out to improve the care-management processes in a particular practice. For example, many high-performing practices use pre-visit planning and pretesting to avoid inefficient visits that don't meet the needs of the patient. A care coordinator might contact an out-of-control diabetic patient who has not visited his or her provider for some time and ask that person to make an appointment. In addition, the care coordinator might arrange for the patient to have an HbA1c test prior to the visit so that the physician can discuss the results with the patient.

This kind of pre-visit planning has been shown to reduce the total amount of work, save time, and improve care.[23] But some providers may feel the approach is not patient-centric, because it requires the patient to come into the office twice or go to a reference lab before his visit. Other doctors expect they might have to order other tests during the encounter; so rather than asking the patient to travel to the lab twice, they'll order the tests at the end of the visit.

What this scenario underlines is the need for continuous quality improvement by care teams trained in Lean principles. Some groups are taking this approach and are finding that it helps them optimize work flows in their own unique environments.

Lean care teams

In the aforementioned study of twenty-three high-performing groups, the researchers observed that the practice from ThedaCare Clinic in Oshkosh, Wisconsin, had raised its clinical and operational performance from last to first place among ThedaCare's twenty-two primary care clinics.

The group attributed this turnaround to systematic work-flow planning using Lean techniques. These methods included identification and elimination of waste through value-stream mapping and process standardization. Clinic site director Kathy Markofski reported, "The team maps out the work flow of a patient visit. We identify wait times, do a root-cause analysis, develop countermeasures, and then quickly reassess with data."[24]

At the Cleveland Clinic, "the physician and clinical staff meet weekly to review data and refine their workflows," the study notes. They look at what went well and what didn't and the changes they need to make to improve the work flows.

Practices that follow Lean principles can benefit from a quality-management committee or a similar entity to supervise the quality-improvement process and make sure that the group is meeting the quality metrics specified in its payer contracts. But this committee should not do the actual work of process improvement.

"They can educate people about what the measures are, and they can be the ones to pull together the quarterly or monthly meetings and share the data so everyone has a common 'line of sight,' which is also a Lean principle," says Karen Handmaker, vice president of population health strategies for Phytel. "But the work is done on the front line, and the care teams build it up from the bottom."

Checklist for Lean Care Management

☐ Make care-team transformation a strategic objective, with assigned leadership and visible executive support.

☐ Create an environment that supports continuous quality improvement.

☐ Form multidisciplinary care teams to share the work of care management.

☐ Map clinical and administrative processes and engage staff in suggesting how they could be improved.

☐ Identify and eliminate waste through value-stream mapping and process standardization.

☐ Reengineer processes to allow each care-team member to perform at the top of his or her license.

☐ Make pre- and post-visit care planning part of the clinical process.

☐ Introduce a quality-management committee to supervise the quality improvement process and track progress and results.

☐ Use automation tools and other technology solutions to reduce waste and improve efficiency—but only after analyzing and reengineering work flows.

Automation in Lean processes

As mentioned earlier, Lean does not require health information technology. One of the earliest and most effective parts of Lean manufacturing, for instance, was the kanban cards used to control and replenish inventory. But by applying health IT and automation tools within a Lean context, organizations can become much more efficient in managing population health.

The majority of primary care practices now have EHRs, which generate data that can be used to improve the quality of care. However, EHRs were not designed as the basis for Lean process improvement.

For example, ThedaCare found that its EHR could not produce a single plan of care for the multiple physicians, nurses, and other professionals who care for patients across the continuum of care, including primary care, specialty care, and the hospital. As a result, multidisciplinary care teams could not use the EHR to coordinate care. Eventually, ThedaCare and its vendor reprogrammed the software to accommodate the single care plan.[25]

Aside from some control-chart and kanban applications, there aren't many off-the-shelf programs designed specifically for the Lean approach in health care, experts say.[26] Some population health management solutions, though, could be adapted to the Lean approach.

Automation tools, for instance, can play an important role in Lean process improvement. These tools cannot fix a broken process; but after a practice has analyzed and reengineered its work flows, it can consider where automation fits in and how it can improve care management processes further. By delegating routine tasks to automation tools, care teams can provide appropriate forms of care management to most of the patient population, while improving their ability to help patients who need human assistance.

Basic automation tools

The first step in this process is to use an analytic application that stratifies the patient population by health risk. For example, a population might be broken down into low-, medium-, and high-risk individuals. This becomes the basis for deciding which automation tools to use with specific patients. The risk-stratification analytics should be applied to a combination of clinical and claims data to get a wide-angle view of patients' health status. Health risk assessment surveys can also be helpful in evaluating patients' health behavior.

Automation tools can be used to link workflows together. For example, a patient-centric registry provides a full picture of all patients, including their health conditions, what services have been provided to them, and when they're due for particular preventive or chronic-care services. Using embedded protocols for recommended care, reports can be run on registry data to reveal patient-care gaps. The program can then send alerts to providers that patients need certain kinds of care, such as mammography or diabetic eye exams, when they come in for their next visit. Another kind of automation tool uses the same registry data and protocols to generate automated messages to patients who need preventive or chronic care. These messages ask them to make appointments with their providers.

A different type of population health application produces work lists that enable care coordinators to prioritize their management of high-risk patients. Instead of having to wade through electronic charts and look at each patient's lab results, recent ER visits, and other relevant data, the care managers can instantly see which patients are at the greatest risk of complications or hospitalization. This type of automation can save a great deal of time and can help the care managers attend to the sickest patients proactively.

A basic assumption of population health management is that many of the patients who have serious health risks are "below the waterline," that is, they haven't yet developed the condition or the exacerbation that will generate high health costs. So to manage population health properly, organizations must target not only high-risk patients but also those with low and medium risks. They must also initiate patient-engagement campaigns to improve the health of those with various chronic conditions and keep healthy patients healthy.

This is an area where automation excels: technology and mobile health-care applications can simultaneously launch hundreds of educational campaigns and other interventions aimed at people in different subcategories. Of course, some patients need human interventions as well, so automation is only part of the mix. If used correctly, automation becomes a member of the care team to which certain tasks are delegated.

"Top-of-license" approach

Earlier, we discussed a care-team model that assigns to every care-team member the work that matches his or her training and expertise. Automation can be part of this "top-of-license" approach. The goal is to assign the right patients to the right staff members or to automation only. With the help of risk stratification, the care team can decide which approach will work best for each individual. A healthy patient might just need automated reminders to maintain wellness and get recommended preventive services. Patients who are at risk of developing a chronic condition might receive automated interventions as well as health coaching from MAs. Nurses and MAs work with patients who have chronic conditions to prevent disease progression and avoid unnecessary complications. And nurse case managers have responsibility for managing high-risk patients with multiple conditions.

Downstream value

The team-based, population health management approach discussed in this chapter confers financial advantages in a value-based reimbursement system. Whether an organization has pay-for-performance, shared savings, or risk contracts, the ability to improve outcomes and lower costs will result in a better bottom line. And health IT is a key component of that capability.

According to the Health Information Management and Systems Society (HIMSS), health IT can create five kinds of value:

- *satisfaction* of patients, providers, staff, and others;
- *treatment/clinical*—patient safety, quality of care, and efficiency;
- *electronic information/data*—use of evidence-based guidelines, data sharing, population health, and quality reporting;
- *prevention/patient education*—improved disease surveillance and patient compliance with therapies; and
- *savings* from improvements, such as reduced days in accounts receivable, patient wait times, and emergency-department admissions.[27]

By eliminating waste and improving care processes, the health IT-enabled Lean approach can provide even more downstream value to payers and accountable care organizations (ACOs). Better ambulatory-care management leads to lower rates of ED visits, hospital admissions, and readmissions. Care-delivery transformation enables primary care physicians to provide more comprehensive care and limit referrals to specialists. And as previously mentioned, the efficient use of care teams also increases practice capacity so providers can see more patients.

Automation tools enable care managers to do more and manage patients better. Practices can use these tools to reach their entire populations, not just those who visit their care providers, which is what population health management is all about. And they can help care-team members practice at the top of their licenses by taking over time-consuming, routine tasks.

"Leaning Out" the Eight Types of Waste in Primary Care

Type of Waste	Lean Definition	Example Solutions
Defects	Errors resulting from omissions, inaccurate information, or mistakes. Errors often require rework and can cause harm.	Use algorithms to evaluate patient-care gaps against evidence-based guidelines and take action to close them with automated patient communications and provider alerts.
Overproduction	Providing more services than needed, including redundant services.	Query integrated patient registry before ordering tests and services for patients.
Waiting	Idle time for the customer or staff member while waiting for needed information, action, or resource.	Build in same-day appointment slots to improve access; redesign visit-preparation process with daily huddles and new roles for care-team members while rooming patients.
Not Fully Utilized	Unused talent, creativity, and skills.	Train medical assistants to do health coaching; delegate or automate nonclinical tasks to maximize use of clinical team members' specialized skills.
Transportation	Moving people, equipment, and supplies takes valuable time and resources.	Do lab testing in the office instead of sending patients to another location.
Inventory	The supply of resources waiting to be consumed by customer demand.	Survey patients to determine best days, times, and locations to hold group education sessions so "supply" matches demand.
Motion	Movement of people or resources while performing tasks.	Colocate physicians and medical assistants in "pods" to eliminate extra steps (walking, messaging) to communicate; utilize automated reporting and alerts to minimize "clicks" and research time.
Excess Processing	Redundant or otherwise non-value-added activities.	Ask patients to update existing information instead of completing new profiles at every visit.

Conclusion

The transformation of health-care delivery requires high-performance care teams. But care teams that include care coordinators and other ancillary professionals are likely to be too expensive for many primary care practices because many important services of care-team members are not reimbursed under most contracts, although this is starting to change.

Value-based reimbursement can justify the higher overhead expense if practices can produce real savings. But to move the needle on cost and quality, practices need to undertake a kind of population health management that's impossible to do with manual methods. Automation tools can enable practices to meet this challenge, while making them more efficient.

Automation alone, however, cannot fix broken processes. One proven way to do that is to use the Lean approach to continuous quality improvement. Lean thinking, coupled with automation tools, can make care teams more efficient and productive, while helping practices deliver value to patients and payers.

Leading health-care organizations are moving in this direction. They will be among the organizations best-suited to succeed in the world of value-based reimbursement.

Automation tools can also enable organizations to engage the majority of their patients in improving their own health. As we explain in the next chapter, patient engagement—a basic tenet of population health management—can achieve only modest success unless providers use all of the technology tools at their disposal to reach patients and persuade them to change their health behavior.

Provider-Led Strategies for Patient Engagement

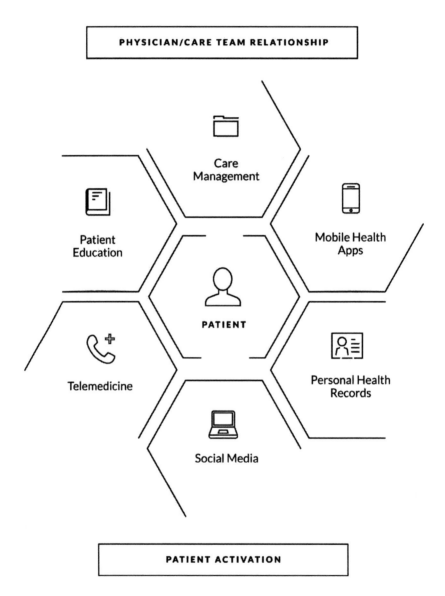

PHYSICIAN/CARE TEAM RELATIONSHIP

Care Management

Patient Education

Mobile Health Apps

PATIENT

Telemedicine

Personal Health Records

Social Media

PATIENT ACTIVATION

Chapter 10

Patient Engagement

- *Introduction*: Patient engagement is essential to improving health outcomes and is therefore an integral part of population health management. Visits to physicians alone are not enough to sustain patient engagement, but the physician-patient relationship is critical to success in this area.

- *How to engage patients*: Patient activation is a formidable challenge. Increasing the patients' knowledge of their condition and building confidence in their ability to change are key factors. Low health literacy, cultural and language differences, and poverty are major barriers to patient engagement.

- *Care management*: The automation of patient outreach can help health-care organizations engage the majority of people in their populations. By combining automation with tools for risk stratification and identification of care gaps, they can also deliver tailored interventions to patients.

- *Patient education*: With a large percentage of people going online for health information, it's natural to use automated, web-based educational materials to teach them more about their conditions. When combined with health coaching and other online communications, this approach can be a powerful tool to increase patient engagement.

- *Telemedicine*: Remote patient monitoring and other forms of telemedicine can also help patients get more involved in their own care, while keeping clinicians apprised of their health status. Numerous studies show the clinical benefits of telemedicine.

- *Mobile health apps:* The proliferation of smartphones and tablet computers offer new routes for physicians to increase patient engagement through apps that promote wellness and better control of chronic conditions.

- *Personal health records:* PHRs have long been viewed as a potentially powerful tool for involving patients in their own care. But so far, PHRs have had fairly low uptake, even by patients with chronic conditions. Physicians must start sharing EHR data with patients and use PHRs in other ways to get patients onboard.

- *Social media:* Social media have had a huge impact on consumers, and the majority of physicians use them in clinical care. But for the most part, they're using these media to obtain information on medical studies and communicate with other health-care professionals, not patients.

As the health-care industry starts to reengineer care delivery to accommodate new reimbursement models, providers on the front lines of change recognize the need for population health management and for increasing patient engagement in their own care. These two approaches are inextricably bound together, because it is impossible to manage the health of a population without getting patients more involved in self-management and the modification of their own risk factors. This chapter discusses the fundamentals of patient engagement and shows how automation tools and web-based care management can facilitate this key process.

Studies demonstrate that patient engagement is essential to improving health outcomes and that the lack of such engagement is a major contributor to preventable deaths. In fact, it is estimated that 40 percent of deaths in the United States are caused by modifiable behavioral issues, such as smoking and obesity. People with chronic diseases take only 50 percent of the prescribed doses of medications, on average. Fifty percent of patients do not follow referral advice, and 75 percent do not keep follow-up appointments.[1]

Many patients are unaware of their risk factors because they have not received recommended screening tests. For example, when a group of 4,000 people were screened for high cholesterol, a government study found, only 40 percent of those who had this condition were aware of it. Even among people who knew they had high cholesterol, only 14.5 percent were taking cholesterol-lowering drugs, and just 6.8 percent had reduced their levels below the goal of 200 mg/dl.[2]

In a study on the impact of eliminating copays on drugs prescribed to heart-attack survivors, the authors noted that rates of adherence to these medications—including statins, beta blockers, ACE inhibitors, and ARBs—ranged from 36 percent to 49 percent.[3] In an accompanying editorial, Lee Goldman, MD, and Arnold M. Epstein, MD, commented, "Perhaps the most sobering findings were both the low baseline adherence and the small improvement in adherence in what should have been a highly motivated group of patients after myocardial infarction."[4]

Visits to physicians alone are insufficient to address the overall compliance problem. "Sporadic contact (such as every six months) with a health care provider is often inadequate to maintain and reinforce complicated lifestyle modifications and pharmacologic regimens," noted Thomas Pearson in a paper on the prevention of cardiovascular disease.[5]

One of the goals of population health management is to maintain continuous contact with patients and to address modifiable health behaviors that may lead to or exacerbate chronic diseases.[6] To be effective, population health management should include a variety of interventions—some of them automated—to keep patients engaged and help them manage their own care between visits.

Physician-patient relationship

It is equally important to recognize that the key to patient engagement is the physician-patient relationship. When a doctor advises a patient to quit smoking, for example, the chance of that person doing so increases by 30 percent.[7] So all patient outreach and intervention efforts must be performed in the name of, or coordinated through, the patient's physician in order to have a strong likelihood of success.

Shared decision making between physicians and patients also increases the probability of improved outcomes,[8] so that must be part of the engagement formula. Although patients vary in their desire to be involved in decision making, one recent study showed that most patients want to participate in major medical decisions.[9]

Shared decision making is a key part of the patient-centered medical home (PCMH), which has been embraced by more and more physician practices and health-care organizations in recent years. In the PCMH, every patient has a personal physician who takes responsibility for his or her care and coordinates referrals across care settings. In addition, the patient is considered part of the care team, and the patient and his or her family can participate in quality improvement at the practice level.[10]

Both in the PCMH and the chronic-care model of disease management, patient engagement is critical. But as every physician knows, it is difficult to motivate many patients to participate in their own health care. What follows are some findings of the recent research on the psychology of patient activation and the interventions that have been shown to engage patients.

How to engage patients

Patient engagement is crucial to improving population health because patients with chronic diseases—who generate 75 percent of health costs— must manage their own conditions most of the time. Care management can help them do that, but they still face a tough challenge, as patient activation expert Judith Hibbard explained:

> Patients with chronic diseases often must follow complex
> treatment regimens, monitor their conditions, make

lifestyle changes, and make decisions about when they need to seek care and when they can handle a problem on their own. Effectively functioning in the role of self-manager, particularly when living with one or more chronic illnesses, requires a high level of knowledge, skill, and confidence.[11]

When patients have the knowledge, skill, and confidence to help manage their own health, Hibbard observed, they do better. "A growing body of evidence shows that patients who are engaged, active participants in their own care have better health outcomes and measurable cost savings," she pointed out.[12]

But it is not easy to activate some patients, either because they are depressed or because they don't believe they are up to the task. According to a report from the Center for Advancing Health, for example, only 30 percent of seniors feel they have the motivation and the skills to participate fully in their own care.[13]

Hibbard and her colleagues characterized patient activation as a developmental process that they broke down into four stages:[14]

- believing the patient role in care is important,
- having the confidence and the knowledge necessary to take action,
- actually taking action to maintain and improve one's health, and
- staying the course even under the stress of adverse life conditions.

In a 2004 study, Hibbard's team looked at whether changes in patient activation led to changes in health behavior in a cohort of people between fifty and seventy years old. The intervention group attended weekly workshops that covered topics related to self-management of care and coping with social isolation. Compared with the control group, the intervention group became more activated initially, but the difference faded after six months. However, individuals in both groups who became more activated had a positive change in a variety of self-management behaviors.[15]

Activation models

How to activate patients to change poor health behavior—which can worsen chronic conditions or cause patients to get sick—has been the subject of considerable research. Here are a few of the approaches that have been tried:

Transtheoretical model. In this approach, care managers or coaches increase awareness of the need for change. Then they motivate patients to make changes and help them make concrete action plans. Later, they assist patients with problem solving and social support, and reinforce maintenance of health behavior changes. The key is to help patients change their self-concept and have them see how social norms support improvements in their health behavior.[16]

Social cognitive theory. The underlying concept of this model is that the more you believe you can do something, the more likely you are to do it. Care managers try to help patients build confidence in their ability to improve health behavior and avoid unhealthy behavior even in stressful conditions. This approach addresses both the psychosocial dynamics influencing healthy behavior and methods for promoting behavior change.[17]

Health belief model. Proponents of this approach argue that many people will change their health behavior if they believe it will help them avoid a negative health outcome. Techniques include defining risk, consequences of risk, and benefits of change; identification of barriers and tips to overcome them; promotion of action through information and reminders; and confidence building through training, guidance, and reinforcement.[18]

Patient Activation Model (PAM). PAM° assessment gauges the knowledge, skills and confidence essential to managing one's own health and healthcare. The PAM assessment segments consumers into one of four progressively higher activation levels. Each level addresses a broad array of self-care behaviors and offers deep insight into the characteristics that drive health activation. A PAM score can also predict healthcare outcomes including medication adherence, ER utilization and hospitalization.

Patients who received PAM coaching tailored to their individual level of activation showed greater improvement in their biometrics and in their adherence to recommended regimens, and showed greater reductions in hospitalizations and in emergency department use than did patients coached in the usual way. [19]

Fogg Behavior Model. According to this theory, three elements must converge at the same moment for a behavior to occur: motivation, ability, and a trigger of some kind. By putting the trigger in the path of someone who wants to change, and showing them that they have the ability to change, it is possible to effect the desired change in behavior. [20]

Obstacles to patient engagement

There are many barriers to patient engagement that go beyond the willingness of patients to take responsibility for self-care or to follow doctors' orders. These include the social and economic environment in which patients must function, cultural factors, the lack of health literacy in a large portion of the population, knowledge deficits, and poor access to health care.

For example, a recent study shows there is a large disparity in patient activation between Hispanic immigrants and white people born in the United States. Some of this disparity—not only between Hispanics and whites, but also between African-Americans and whites—has to do with social and economic differences, the study found. But in the case of Hispanics, cultural and language barriers also play an important role in the disparity.[21]

The lack of health literacy is a major obstacle across the US population. More than 90 million adults have low health literacy, meaning they have difficulty understanding and using health information.[22] Educational materials often are not written at a level that people can easily grasp and make use of—a situation that is exacerbated when a patient's primary language is not English.

Finally, many people simply lack good access to health care. They may not have a regular primary care physician; and even if they do have one, it may be difficult to get an appointment, to take time off from work, or to find transportation to see the doctor. Additionally, some patients cannot afford the tests or medications that their physician orders, especially if they lack insurance.

Population health management cannot overcome all of these obstacles to patient engagement. But the automation of care management and care coordination can significantly improve the odds that the majority of patients can be actively engaged in managing their own care. This can be done in several domains, including care management, patient education, and interventions that utilize a variety of new technologies.

Care management

Most physicians do not have enough time to keep track of all of their patients, let alone reach out to them between visits. Moreover, there are many lower-level clinical tasks that can be performed by nonphysicians or can be automated. So in any organization focused on population health, a care team does the day-to-day work of caring for and engaging the patient.

In some health-care organizations, care managers focus mainly on telephonic management of high-risk patients who may be admitted to the hospital or go to the emergency department unless their urgent needs are met. This is an important task of the care team, but it is only one component of population health management. Of the patients who generate the highest costs in a given year, less than 30 percent would have been included in the high-risk category the year prior.[23] So, an organization that hopes to improve the quality and lower the cost of care must pay attention to its entire population.

Maintaining continuous contact with every patient in a practice, however, is a task that exceeds the capability of even the largest health-care organizations if they use only manual processes. Care managers are expensive, and the number of patients they can supervise is limited. To expand their reach and the influence of physicians on their patients, some degree of automation is required.

Patient outreach

For example, many patients have gaps in their preventive and chronic care. In some cases, this is because they haven't visited the practice in a long time. In other cases, they haven't been told they need these services during office visits, or they haven't complied with their physician's recommendations.

Some practices try to contact patients with care gaps between visits. But even if a practice has a good system for identifying these patients, manual outreach is prohibitively costly in terms of staff time, phone, and mailing costs. So, this is usually a hit-or-miss process, and it is not scalable to larger groups.

New automation tools can facilitate this part of the patient-engagement process and ensure outreach to all patients who need services. Using data extracted from a practice management system or an electronic health record, these solutions build patient registries and use clinical protocols to trigger messaging to patients who have an existing care gap and need to make an appointment with their physician. Frequently, this messaging results in patients getting back in touch with their physicians after a long absence.

A study at Prevea Health, a large multispecialty group in Green Bay, Wisconsin, showed that automated outreach to noncompliant patients with diabetes or hypertension increases the likelihood that those patients will make office visits and get the care they need. The study concluded, "An automated identification and outreach program can be an effective means to supplement existing practice patterns to ensure that patients with chronic conditions in need of care receive the necessary treatment."[24]

Risk stratification

As mentioned earlier, the majority of high-cost patients today had a much lower risk of generating high costs a year ago. So, organizations that want to do population health management must adopt techniques to identify patients who are likely to become high risk and prioritize care management of those patients (see chapter 6).

Some health insurers are giving accountable care organizations predictive modeling software—similar to the programs their actuaries use—to accomplish that task.[25] But it is also possible to do risk stratification—while also increasing patient engagement—by asking patients to complete online health risk assessments, just as many employers and health plans do.[26] Though patients resist filling out long forms, practices can break up HRAs into smaller, bite-size chunks about specific areas of a patient's health behavior, such as diet, exercise, or smoking.

HRAs enable organizations to classify patients by their health conditions, health behaviors, and functional status. This helps providers spot patients who may become high-risk and gives them data for analyzing their patient population. In addition, some HRAs measure stages of patient activation—something that Hibbard recommends. "This would enable early intervention with patients who lack the skills to self-manage before they inevitably move to a higher health-risk group," she noted in a *Health Affairs* paper.[27]

It's important to remember, however, that HRAs or any other type of patient-entered data can supply only part of the information needed for accurate risk stratification. Analytics that use claims data and clinical data are needed to round out the picture for each patient.

Patient education

The research on patient activation shows that patients feel more confident about managing their health condition when they have more knowledge about it. Today, many patients go online for this information. In a September 2012 survey by the Pew Research Center, 72 percent of adult Internet users said they'd sought answers to their health questions online in the past year, and 35 percent said they'd gone online to figure out what medical condition they or another person might have.[28] Another survey shows that Americans are more likely to seek health information on the web than from doctors, pharmacists, or nurses.[29] Still, 71 percent of patients consult physicians or other health professionals when they have a serious health problem.[30]

Online patient education materials may be multimedia and interactive—a big improvement over the paper handouts that many practices still use. When patients view some of these programs, they can ask questions and receive answers online. One vendor of online education services even allows physicians to see whether patients have reviewed the materials they were asked to read or view. Such materials are available both for postsurgical care and the care of chronic conditions.[31]

When combined with automated patient communications, these online educational materials can be powerful tools to motivate patients. Physicians can put in a standing order for particular education pieces to be directed automatically to patients at various points in the care process. Such an approach relieves the burden on practice staff of ensuring that patients receive the proper information at the appropriate time.

Health coaching has also been shown to improve patient outcomes, and there is some evidence that online coaching has similar results.[32,33] The latest digital coaching tools, which start with health risk assessments, can help patients improve their health behaviors by losing weight, eating better, or exercising more, for example.[34]

To have the desired effect, these automated education and health-coaching tools must be tailored to the target population. They must not only be condition-specific, but they must also be written in consumer-friendly language. They must be designed to address health literacy and language barriers, or they will fail. [35]

Telemedicine

The use of remote patient monitoring and alerting in chronic-disease management dates back to the late 1990s.[36] Since then, telemonitoring devices have become more sophisticated and less expensive, and the ability to transmit data has grown exponentially. The main obstacle to faster growth of telemonitoring is the health-care reimbursement system, which still does not compensate physicians for non-visit care in most cases. That barrier, too, is expected to disappear as accountable care becomes the new paradigm.

Telemonitoring helps care teams extend their reach, and it engages patients in their own care. It has also been shown to improve outcomes when combined with active care management. According to a 2004 study of telemonitoring in diabetes care, for instance, "prompting follow-up procedures, computerized insulin therapy adjustment using home glucose records, remote feedback, and counseling have documented benefits in improving diabetes-related outcomes."[37]

In a 2007 report, the Agency for Healthcare Research and Quality (AHRQ) surveyed the literature on the impact of what it called "consumer health informatics [CHI] applications," which would now be called telemedicine or telehealth.[38] The majority of the studies evaluated interactive, web-based applications or web-based, tailored educational applications. Fifteen percent of the studies looked at computer-generated tailored feedback applications, and 8 percent evaluated interactive computer programs and personal monitoring devices.

The meta-analysis found that the CHI interventions improved self-management, knowledge of health conditions, adherence to treatments, and health behavior. Some of the studies evaluated clinical outcomes for cancer, diabetes, mental health, diet, exercise and physical activity, asthma, COPD, breast cancer, Alzheimer's disease, arthritis, back pain, aphasia, HIV/AIDS, headache, obesity, and pain. "Over 80 percent of studies found significant influence of CHI applications on at least one clinical outcome," the report concluded.

More recent studies confirm the benefits of telemedicine. A 2008 study by the Veterans Health Administration (VHA) found that the VHA's telemedicine program reduced hospital-bed days by 25 percent and hospital admissions by 19 percent for a cohort of 17,000 participating patients.[39] A 2012 study of telemedicine in a California care-coordination program found that it reduced mortality rates for patients with congestive heart failure by 57 percent over three years.[40]

Mobile health apps

In recent years, the number of people using smartphones, tablets, and other web-connected mobile devices has exploded. According to the Pew Research Center, 58 percent of US adults now own smartphones, and 42 percent have tablet computers.[41]

The rise of mobile communications has been accompanied by rapid growth in the number of health-related applications designed for mobile devices. While many of these are intended for professionals, the bulk of them are aimed at consumers. These applications range from symptom checkers and apps that measure vital signs to programs that help users find "quality"-evaluated doctors and hospitals.[42] The latest iPhones and iPads also have "video-chat" features that physicians can use to examine patients remotely.[43]

The mobile health apps that have the greatest potential in population health management are those linked to care management. In a 2011 study, for example, a mobile, web-based self-management patient coaching system was shown to help patients with diabetes reduce their HbA1c levels more than a control group that received usual care.[44] Another study showed that mobile alerts to diabetic patients using glucometers with smartphones were as effective in lowering HbA1c as an Internet-based glucose-monitoring system.[45]

Personal health records

The value of personal health records (PHRs) has been debated and continues to be uncertain. But in large health-care organizations like Kaiser Permanente and Group Health Cooperative, where PHRs are linked to EHRs, millions of patients are using PHRs to view parts of their medical record, see lab results, request prescription refills, schedule appointments, and e-mail their physicians.[46] Patients at the Palo Alto Medical Foundation who had PHRs indicated that these tools made them feel like part of the medical team and kept them in closer touch with their providers.[47]

In a study of the use of health IT in patient-centered medical homes, David W. Bates and Asaf Bitton noted that PHRs can increase patient engagement and self-efficacy, but that they have low uptake by patients, especially those who are chronically ill. One reason, they said, is that current PHRs have serious limitations; for example, many do not include clinical data from EHRs and other sources.[48]

To remedy these defects, they argued, physicians must overcome their reluctance to share EHR data with patients, and interfaces must be improved to make it easy for patients to download clinical data. In addition, PHRs should have the capability to communicate online with care teams and track vital signs such as weight, blood pressure, and blood sugar. There should also be a mechanism for care managers to provide feedback when a patient's indicators are worrisome, the authors said.

Another study maintained that the potential of PHRs will not be realized until they integrate a wide range of patient data that go beyond the EHR in a particular practice or organization. In addition, the paper said, such integrated PHRs must include a range of tools to help consumers apply the data to self-management.

> The data elements within an electronic PHR record alone are not sufficient to realize improvements that can be considered transformative. Significant value will be realized only when PHRs incorporate systems, tools, and

other resources that leverage the data in the record and enable consumers to play a more active role in their health and health care.[49]

Social media

Social media such as Facebook, Twitter, and LinkedIn are having a huge impact on consumers. Some people spend more time on social media than they do on all other Internet sites combined. From a logical viewpoint, it would seem that patient-engagement strategies should include the use of social media.

But physicians and their patients use different social media, and doctors are not eager to communicate with patients via Facebook or Twitter.

A 2012 survey showed that a quarter of physicians used social media daily in their clinical work. Sixty-one percent of respondents did so at least once a week, and 58 percent found social media was beneficial and improved patient care.[50]

Another study discovered that 67 percent of doctors employ social media for professional purposes, but their top destinations are professional sites and LinkedIn. The majority of doctors use Facebook in their personal lives, but only 15 percent use it in health care. And while a third of physicians have received invitations to "friend" their patients, 75 percent of those doctors declined to do so.[51]

The biggest reason for physicians to avoid using Facebook and Twitter for professional purposes is the fear of breaching professional confidentiality online. In addition, some doctors are afraid of learning things about patients that the patient has chosen not to disclose, such as recreational drug use. And many doctors prefer to keep their personal and professional lives separate.[52]

Nevertheless, physicians and care teams can refer patients with specific conditions to online communities that provide education and mutual support to people with those conditions. That would certainly increase patient engagement. But before they do so, doctors would be well-advised to check out these sites to make sure that they're providing reliable, objective information.

Conclusion

Patient engagement is vital to quality improvement, better patient outcomes, and population health management. To improve patient engagement, organizations must reach out to every patient, using the techniques that have been shown to motivate patients to participate in their own health care.

Care teams provide the non-visit, continuous care that is essential to population health management. They are also responsible for promoting patient engagement between visits. But care managers who use manual processes cannot intervene with every patient. That effort requires the use of health information and communication tools that automate the process so that care managers can devote themselves to the patients who need the most attention.

Besides automating care management, the latest technologies enable organizations to analyze population data and stratify patients by risk. Based on that information, they can design engagement strategies tailored to particular subgroups of patients.

Other new technologies, ranging from telemonitoring and mobile health to PHRs and social media, can be employed to increase patient engagement. But to be effective, they must be linked with provider-led care management, and they must invoke the power and influence of the doctor-patient relationship.

By combining all of these techniques, health-care organizations can provide truly patient-centered care. When patients are fully engaged in their own health care, they will have better outcomes, and the growth in health costs will start to abate.

An important aspect of patient engagement that we haven't explored yet is post-discharge care. Hospitals have recently become very focused on this kind of care, because of Medicare's penalties for preventable readmissions. The final chapter in this book takes a close look at the implications of post-discharge care, the challenges to ensuring that patients receive proper follow-up, and the role that information technology can play in making that happen.

Chapter 11

Automated Post-Discharge Care

- *Introduction:* Readmissions, which affect nearly a fifth of Medicare patients discharged from the hospital, are more numerous than they should be because of the fragmentation of our health-care system. Various government programs have been established to address this problem.
- *Gaps in care transitions:* Among the reasons for preventable readmissions are poor preparation of patients in the hospital, poor handovers to ambulatory-care providers, and a lack of hospital follow-up after discharge.
- *Best practices:* Academic experts have identified several approaches that can reduce readmissions. Examined here are the Institute for Healthcare Improvement's (IHI's) recommendations, the Coleman Care Transitions Intervention, and the Naylor Transitional Care Model.
- *Automation:* While these approaches have proved successful with some patients and subpopulations, they can't be applied to all discharged patients because they rely on one-to-one case management. To reduce readmissions further, health-care organizations should employ automated methods of following up with patients and making sure their needs are met.

Readmissions are a major problem in US health care. Nearly one in five Medicare patients discharged from the hospital returns there within thirty days,[1] and between 50 percent and 75 percent of those readmissions are considered preventable.[2] Medicare pays about $17 billion annually for 2.5 million rehospitalizations of its beneficiaries, and other payers spend roughly the same amount every year for all readmissions of non-Medicare patients.[3]

The immediate cause of a readmission is usually a rapid deterioration in the patient's condition, related to the patient's primary diagnosis or comorbidities. But in a broader sense, it can be attributed to systemic failures that begin in the hospital and continue in the fragmented health-care settings that patients move through after discharge.

In a typical scenario, patients receive inadequate preparation for discharge, the handover from the hospital to their outpatient providers is poorly handled, and patients and their family caregivers are left to cope on their own with medical issues that they don't understand.[4] In fact, only about half of discharged patients follow up with their primary-care physicians after they leave the hospital, and those who don't are much more likely to be readmitted than those who do see a doctor.[5]

New Government Incentives

Until recently, some hospitals took the attitude that their responsibility for care ended when the patient walked (or was wheeled) out the door. Other facilities have used a variety of techniques to reduce readmissions, with mixed results. But new government incentives, plus a rising awareness of the need to improve patient safety, are forcing hospitals to place an increased emphasis on discharge planning and post-acute care.

Front and center are the Centers for Medicare and Medicaid's (CMS's) regulations on preventable readmissions. Since October 1, 2012, hospitals with "excessive" readmissions—rehospitalizations that are significantly higher than expected—have lost a percentage of their Medicare reimbursement across the board. In FY 2013, the decrease was up to 1 percent of reimbursement; that penalty increased to 2 percent in 2014 and will rise to 3 percent in 2015.[6]

In the first year of this program, CMS examined thirty-day readmission rates for patients with heart failure, acute myocardial infarction, and pneumonia—three of the leading conditions for which patients are readmitted. Beginning in FY 2015, CMS will also scrutinize readmissions for an acute exacerbation of chronic obstructive pulmonary disease (COPD), elective total hip arthroplasty, and total knee arthroplasty.[7]

This program has already had some effect. In the last quarter of 2012, the all-cause readmission rate for Medicare dropped to 17.8 percent from the historical rate of 19 percent. That represented about 70,000 fewer readmissions than expected.[8]

CMS has also launched other programs that might contribute to lower readmission rates. To begin with, the agency plans to spend $500 million—or half of the $1 billion earmarked in the Affordable Care Act for improving patient safety—to help hospitals and their community partners decrease readmissions over a five-year period ending in 2016. Through the government-sponsored Partnership for Patients, CMS is paying these "community-based organizations" a set amount per discharge for managing Medicare beneficiaries at high risk for readmission.[9]

Two other CMS initiatives authorized by the health reform law are also designed to cut readmissions: payment bundling and accountable care organizations.

Under CMS's bundling demonstration, which started in April 2013, providers may choose among four different options. These choices include retrospective bundled payments to hospitals, physicians, and other providers for acute care only; hospital care plus post-acute care for a specified period; and post-acute care only. The fourth option involves a lump-sum prospective payment for hospital care plus readmissions that occur during the thirty days after discharge.[10]

The Medicare Shared-Savings Program (MSSP) for accountable care organizations (ACOs), which began in 2012, is also expected to have an effect. ACOs have a strong incentive to cut readmissions in order to generate savings that they can share.[11]

Nevertheless, it's difficult for health-care organizations to decrease readmissions significantly in our fragmented, uncoordinated health-care system. While most of the levers of improvement are known, reengineering inpatient processes and engaging patients and outpatient providers remain challenging.

Fortunately, new applications of health information technology now offer inexpensive ways to automate post-acute-care processes. These solutions, which are discussed later in this chapter, can raise the effectiveness of care managers, improve the communications between inpatient and outpatient providers, and make it easier for patients and caregivers to absorb and apply the knowledge required for self-management of complex conditions.

Gaps in care transitions

The literature on care-transition problems shows there are five main areas that contribute to preventable readmissions:

- poor preparation for discharge,
- patients' low health literacy and comprehension,
- failure or inability of patients to see physicians for follow-up after discharge,
- lack of hospital follow-up, and
- lack of communication between inpatient and outpatient providers.

Readmissions occur, by definition, after a patient has left the hospital. Yet the foundation for post-acute care is laid during the hospital stay—and that preparation is often inadequate. "The hospital discharge process is characterized by fragmented, nonstandardized, and haphazard care," note Brian Jack, an expert on hospital reengineering, and his colleagues.[12]

Nurses and first-year residents are often placed in charge of discharges. These staffers have many other duties and may relegate discharges to a lower priority. Making matters worse, there are no clear lines of authority. As a result, the system sets these individuals up to fail and creates a dangerous situation for patients.

A prime safety issue cited by many experts is missing or inadequate medication reconciliation at the time of discharge. The medications that patients received in the hospital are often discontinued at discharge, while the drugs they were taking before they were admitted may or may not be resumed. Dosages may also change.[13]

The Joint Commission has identified medication reconciliation as a key requirement for ensuring patient safety.[14] The Institute for Healthcare Improvement also cites medication reconciliation as an opportunity to reduce readmissions.[15] So this is clearly an area where hospitals could contribute to lower rehospitalization rates.

Poor educational techniques

Another challenge is getting patients to understand what will be required of them after discharge. In one study, for example, 78 percent of patients discharged from the ER did not understand their diagnosis, their ER treatment, home-care instructions, or warning signs of when to return to the hospital.[16]

Providers are partly responsible for this lack of comprehension. Physicians or nurses may rush through their instructions and not encourage patients to ask questions. They may not use the proven "teach-back" method of having patients restate the instructions in their own words. And they may not realize that because of a patient's cognitive issues, his or her family caregiver is the one who needs to receive the instructions.[17]

Another big—and underappreciated—problem is the low health literacy of the US population. Roughly 90 million Americans—nearly half of the adult population—have low functional literacy.[18] "Such patients typically have difficulty reading and understanding medical instructions, medication labels, and appointment slips," according to one study.[19]

What this means is that both oral and written instructions must be couched in terms that someone with fairly little formal education can understand. It also means that many patients require post-discharge communications to ensure that they are adhering to their medication regimens, following up with their outpatient physicians, and looking for danger signs in their own conditions.

Poor handovers

Another glaring deficiency in post-acute transitions of care is the inadequate communications between inpatient and outpatient providers. Here are a few statistics that underline the chaotic state of these communications:

- Direct communication between hospital physicians and primary care physicians occurs in only 3 to 20 percent of cases.
- Only 12 to 34 percent of doctors have received hospital discharge summaries by the time patients make their first post-discharge visits. The range rises to only 51 to 77 percent after four weeks, affecting the quality of care in about a quarter of follow-up visits.[20]
- Approximately 40 percent of patients have pending test results at the time of discharge, and 10 percent of those require some action; yet in the majority of cases, outpatient physicians are unaware of these results.[21]

Other studies have found that discharge summaries often fail to provide basic information about hospital visits. Some summaries never even reach the primary care doctors who are caring for discharged patients.[22]

While ambulatory-care physicians may be shooting in the dark when they see a recently discharged patient, at least they may know something about the patient's history, and they can find out what medications they're on. All of that works to the patient's advantage. But many discharged patients don't or can't make an appointment to see a doctor within a week of discharge. If the patient is at high risk of complications and deterioration, they should be seen within twenty-four hours, but often this doesn't happen.

Best practices

A great deal of research has been done on the best methods for reducing readmissions. In this section, we will focus on the Institute for Healthcare Improvement's (IHI's) recommendations, the Coleman Care Transitions Intervention, and the Naylor Transitional Care Model.

Other resources for health-care organizations include the BOOST program of the Society of Hospital Medicine,[23] the Care Transitions Performance Measurement Set of the Physician Consortium for Performance Improvement,[24] and the Transitions of Care Consensus Policy Statement of the American College of Physicians and five other specialty societies.[25]

IHI's Patient-Centered Approach

IHI, a Boston-based nonprofit organization that has led two transitions-of-care initiatives, recommends that health-care organizations create "cross-continuum" teams that involve all community stakeholders. It advises institutions to use a patient-centered approach that looks at post-discharge care through a patient's eyes. By doing "deep dives" into several patient histories, IHI says, and finding out why the patients were readmitted, it's possible to understand where the entire process falls short and begin to fix it.[26]

Specifically, IHI recommends:

- focusing on the patient's journey over time across care settings,
- making discharge preparations early,
- redesigning health-education materials using health literacy principles,

- providing intensive care-management services for high-risk patients,
- making sure that patients have follow-up appointments with physicians, and
- improving communications between inpatient and outpatient providers.

The key changes that hospitals need to make, says IHI, are:

- enhanced assessment of post-discharge needs,
- effective teaching and learning by patients or caregivers,
- real-time handover communications, and
- assurance of post-hospital follow-up.[27]

Coleman Care Transitions Intervention

Eric Coleman, MD, a geriatrician at the University of Colorado Health Sciences Center, and his colleagues have created a Care Transitions Intervention (CTI) model that emphasizes the use of a transition coach.[28,29] Recognizing that patients and their caregivers are key parts of the post-discharge care team, the transition coach visits the patient in the hospital and again at home and makes three follow-up phone calls. The coach teaches the patients and caregivers, helps them develop self-management skills, and assesses their learning. While some coaches are nurses, studies have shown that people with a wide variety of backgrounds can perform this function.

Overall, the CTI supports patients in four areas:

- making sure patients and caregivers can manage their medications;
- giving patients personal health records to facilitate communications with providers and promote continuity of care;
- scheduling, preparing for, and completing follow-up visits with physicians; and
- understanding danger signs for their conditions and knowing how to respond to them.

Studies have shown that the CTI approach reduces the chances of rehospitalization by 40 to 50 percent.[30-31] According to a California Healthcare Foundation report, more than 130 hospitals across the United States have adopted the CTI model.[32]

Naylor Transitional Care Model

Mary Naylor, PhD, RN, and her colleagues at the University of Pennsylvania have developed another approach for decreasing readmissions. Their model involves care coordination by a transitional-care nurse, who generally has advanced practice training.[33]

Following evidence-based protocols, the nurse care manager visits the patient daily during his or her hospital stay; visits the patient at home during the first twenty-four hours after discharge and then weekly during the first month; telephones the patient weekly; implements a care plan that is continually reassessed in consultation with the patient, the caregiver, and the patient's primary care physician; and continues calling the patient monthly after the initial two-month period.

Randomized controlled trials have shown that the Naylor model reduces all-cause readmission rates; increases patient satisfaction, function, and quality of life; and decreases overall health-care costs. In one study, the model reduced the number of readmissions at six months by 36 percent, and costs by 39 percent.[34]

The literature on the efficacy of post-discharge phone calls has shown mixed results. But in one study, 19 percent of patients experienced medication-related issues that were resolved with post-discharge calls.[35] In another study, 35 percent of patients who received calls needed significant referral and aftercare instructions.[36] This evidence points to the need to reach out to the whole population of discharged patients, while stratifying patients in order to increase the efficacy of these phone calls and of care management in general.

Automation

The approaches outlined above have been shown to work with certain kinds of patients, and they can also be cost-effective with particular subpopulations. But without the aid of automation, most organizations cannot afford to use these high-touch approaches to reach all patients who have been discharged from the hospital. Moreover, their approach to patient education is not as cost-effective as it could be, because it relies on one-to-one communications between patients or caregivers and coaches or nurses.

The existing models are also labor-intensive in other respects. The coaches and nurse case managers in the Coleman and Naylor models can handle only a limited number of patients. And while human contact is essential in high-risk cases, automated approaches can perform many of the basic tasks required to support moderate- and low-risk patients during the post-discharge transition.

New automation tools can greatly facilitate the range of best practices designed to improve post-discharge care and reduce readmissions. Among the areas where automation can pay off in higher quality and lower costs are:

- risk stratification of patients,
- post-discharge communications with patients,
- patient education and engagement, and
- closing provider communication loops.

Assessing patient risk

Some patients who are at high risk for readmission can be identified in the hospital. Certain conditions, such as congestive heart failure, make readmission likely; but in many cases, comorbidities are responsible for rehospitalization.[37] So some patients who are not obvious candidates for readmission may slip through the cracks. Other factors, such as adverse drug events because of poor or no medication reconciliation, can also lead to unexpected ER visits or readmissions.[38]

Ideally, hospitals should use predictive modeling to identify high-risk patients who are likely to be readmitted if they don't receive appropriate care after discharge. Utilized widely by managed-care plans, predictive-modeling software analyzes hospital data, claims data on utilization and comorbidities, and patient surveys to stratify patients by risk level.

During the critical twenty-four to seventy-two hours after discharge, an automated phone assessment can be used to measure the satisfaction of discharged patients with their care, while gathering data on their risk factors. This information allows a computer program to calculate a risk score. Based on that and on answers to condition-specific questions, alerts about high-risk patients can be transmitted to hospital care managers or triage nurses.

In addition, patients receiving automated calls may choose to be transferred to a hospital nurse help line or a call center if they prefer to speak to someone immediately about their concerns instead of receiving a subsequent callback. Concerns may include worsening conditions, discharge or medication instruction questions, help scheduling appointments, or other care-related concerns.

If a patient has been identified in the hospital as high-risk, a nurse or transition coach should follow up with that patient at home or in the next care setting. Home telemonitoring may also be indicated, particularly for patients with heart failure. Signals from monitoring equipment alert care managers when the patient's condition deteriorates. But for low- or medium-risk patients, the automated-survey approach can establish whether the patient needs further professional assistance.

Moreover, the system can tell the hospital staff whether or not the patient has a follow-up appointment with a physician. And if it is connected with an outpatient registry, it can supplement hospital data with medical histories from integrated primary care systems.

Patient education and engagement

Automation can also provide better, more consistent patient education that overcomes health literacy problems and ensures that patients understand the information they're receiving. This is an enormous opportunity to help patients increase their confidence and their ability to do self-management, while reducing the amount of time and labor required to boost patients to that level.

Web-based, audiovisual educational materials are available, and some of them even provide feedback to providers so that they can see whether patients have viewed the materials.[39] But traditional programs lack the ability to test the patients on what they've learned and make sure they're applying that knowledge to their own care. Digital coaching tools can fill this gap and help patients manage their conditions as much as they can on their own.[40]

Connecting providers to each other

As the statistics cited earlier show, the communication between hospital physicians and ambulatory-care doctors is generally subpar. There are a number of reasons for this, including a shortage of time, the difficulty of reaching outpatient providers, and the inherent problems of phone and fax communications.

The patient-outreach system described earlier can help close the communication loop in one significant respect: if ambulatory-care providers are using the same system to contact patients with preventive and chronic-care needs, that service can also be used to notify primary care physicians and outpatient care managers when patients in their panels are admitted to the hospital and after they are discharged. This alone would fill a significant communication void.

The Physician Consortium for Performance Improvement and an article in the *Journal of Hospital Medicine*[41,42] both recommend providing a transition summary to primary care doctors within twenty-four hours, rather than waiting for discharge summaries to be prepared and transmitted. Such a summary, which could be communicated by phone, fax, or e-mail, would include discharge diagnosis, medications, procedure results, pending test results, follow-up arrangements, and suggested next steps.[43]

The use of EHRs could speed the delivery of these summaries; but as one observer notes, hospitals and ambulatory-care practices frequently use different systems that are incompatible.[44] In the future, health information exchanges may overcome this barrier. Meanwhile, health-care systems could investigate the use of the Direct Project protocol to "push" information from one EHR to another.[45]

Conclusion

By preventing readmissions, health-care organizations could improve patient health and safety, while responding to new government incentives and penalties. A patient-centered, automated approach is the most efficient and cost-effective way to make sure that all patients who have been discharged are properly taken care of. But such a model must be judiciously combined with high-touch care management to address the needs of high-risk patients appropriately.

Conclusion

In the decade that followed the managed-care assault of the 1990s, health care largely slid back into its traditional volume-based approach to care delivery. But today, everything is changing at warp speed to accommodate the rapid growth of value-based reimbursement. Health-care systems that fail to keep up will eventually go out of business or be absorbed by nimbler, more-efficient organizations.

Health care is a huge industry, and there is a vast divide between the leaders of the second managed-care revolution and those who are struggling to figure it out. In the latter camp are the majority of health-care organizations, which still don't entirely understand population health management or the health IT applications designed to support it.

External forces are beginning to change this situation, however. As discussed in the last chapter, Medicare penalties for excessive readmissions are pushing hospitals to work more closely with discharged patients, their physicians, and post-acute-care providers. Health-care systems are also starting to collect data and analyze them in ways they've never done before. It's likely that as these organizations start focusing on other areas of quality improvement, they'll use analytic and automation tools to scale their efforts to the whole patient population.

The growing competition among vendors of PHM software, as well as EHR vendors that are moving into this space, should also lead to greater efforts to educate providers about population health management. Some of these companies are already beginning to offer consulting services and educational tools to help providers get to first base.

Once health-care organizations have grasped the basics of PHM and how to make their data actionable, they will be ready to reengineer themselves. First they will build care teams that enable clinicians to operate at the top of their licenses. Then they will apply analytic and automation applications to facilitate care management, increase efficiency, and scale PHM to the entire population. Some organizations will also adopt a Lean approach to improve their work processes. Part of Lean thinking is to use information technology to automate as many routine tasks as possible.

Meanwhile, the current trend of telehealth and remote patient monitoring will continue to grow. Technology-enabled care delivery will evolve to the point where much that is now done in physician offices, hospitals, and outpatient settings can be done at home. Patients will use mobile apps to communicate with their providers wherever they are, to keep them apprised of changes in their health condition, and to improve their own health behavior so that they can maintain their health. Health risk assessments, functional status surveys, and other types of patient-generated data will also become commonplace. Sophisticated algorithms will filter all of this information so that providers see only the data that they need to respond to.

In the end, population health management depends on using sophisticated information technology to support both patient engagement and medical decision making. Data are oxygen, and the successful organizations will be those that have the best data and know how to use them to create the best outcomes.

Endnotes

Introduction

1. Anne B. Martin, Micah Hartman, Lekha Whittle, Aaron Catlin, and the National Health Expenditure Accounts Team, "National Health Spending in 2012: Rate of Health Spending Growth Remained Low for The Fourth Consecutive Year," *Health Affairs* 33, no. 1 (2014): 67–77.
2. Institute of Medicine, *Crossing the Quality Chasm: A New Health System for the 21st Century.* Washington, DC: National Academy Press, 2001, 3–4.
3. Joseph R. Swedish, "Opening Keynote Address at the Business Health Agenda 2014," March 5, 2014, 3, accessed at http://www.wellpoint.com/prodcontrib/groups/wellpoint/documents/wlp_assets/pw_e213326.pdf.
4. Emily Berry, "United to Attach Performance Conditions to More Doctors' Pay," *American Medical News*, Feb. 29, 2012, accessed at http://www.amednews.com/article/20120229/business/302299997/8/.
5. Aetna Accountable Care Solutions, http://www.aetnaacs.com.
6. Centers for Medicare and Medicaid Services (CMS), Medicare Shared Savings Program, http://www.cms.gov/Medicare/Medicare-Fee-for-Service-Payment/sharedsavingsprogram/index.html?redirect=/.
7. Robinson & Cole Health Law Pulse, "Final Regulations on Accountable Care Organizations Released," accessed at http://www.rc.com/publications/upload/2070.pdf.
8. CMS, "Hospital Value-Based Purchasing," accessed at http://www.cms.gov/Medicare/Quality-Initiatives-Patient-Assessment-Instruments/

hospital-value-based-purchasing/index.html?redirect=/
hospital-value-based-purchasing/.

9. Ken Terry, "VBMs: Coming Soon to Either Increase or Lower Your Income," *Medscape*, Feb. 6, 2014, accessed at http://www.medscape.com/viewarticle/820050_1.

10. NCQA, "The Future of Patient-Centered Medical Homes," accessed at http://www.ncqa.org/Portals/0/Public%20Policy/2014%20Comment%20Letters/The_Future_of_PCMH.pdf.

11. Thomas H. Lee and Toby Cosgrove, "Engaging Doctors in the Health Care Revolution," *Harvard Business Review* (June 2014), accessed at http://hbr.org/2014/06/engaging-doctors-in-the-health-care-revolution/ar/1.

12. Trust for America's Health, "F as in Fat: How Obesity Threatens America's Future," August 2013, accessed at http://healthyamericans.org/report/108/.

13. CMS, "Stage 1 vs. Stage 2 Comparison Table for Eligible Professionals," August 2012, accessed at https://www.cms.gov/Regulations-and-Guidance/Legislation/EHRIncentivePrograms/Downloads/Stage1vsStage2CompTablesforEP.pdf.

14. Health IT Policy Committee, Meaningful Use Workgroup, "Stage 3 Draft Recommendations," March 11, 2014, accessed at http://www.healthit.gov/FACAS/sites/faca/files/HITPC_MUWG_Stage3_Recs_2014-03-11_v6_0.pdf.

15. Phytel, Phytel Outreach™, accessed at http://www3.phytel.com/solutions/population-health-management-systems/proactive-patient-outreach.aspx.

16. K. F. Foreman, K. M. Stockl, L. B. Le, Eric Fisk, Sameer M. Shah, Heidi C. Lew, Brian K. Solow, and Bradford S. Curtis, "Impact of a Text Messaging Pilot Program on Patient Medication Adherence," *Clinical Therapeutics,* Accepted April 12, 2012. Published online May 3, 2012, doi:10.1016/j.clinthera.2012.04.007, http://www.clinicaltherapeutics.com/article/S0149-2918(12)00265-2/abstract.

17. Anna-Lisa Silvestre, Valerie M. Sue, and Jill Y. Allen, "If You Build It, Will They Come? The Kaiser Permanente Model of Online Health Care," *Health Affairs* 28, no. 2 (March/April 2009): 334–344, accessed at http://content.healthaffairs.org/content/28/2/334.abstract?sid=e9b8b36d-7acc-495f-b207-0a0e76b917aa.

18. Ken Terry, "Strategy: How Mobility, Apps and BYOD Will Transform Healthcare," July 1, 2012, accessed at http://reports.informationweek.com/abstract/105/8914/Healthcare/strategy-how-mobility-apps-and-byod-will-transform-healthcare.html.

19. Institute for Health Technology Transformation, "Lean IT: Making Healthcare More Efficient," Sept. 20, 2013, accessed at http://ihealthtran.com/wordpress/2013/09/iht²-report-lean-it-making-healthcare-more-efficient/.

20. Surescripts, "Medication History Ambulatory," accessed at http://surescripts.com/products-and-services/medication-network-services/medication-history-ambulatory.

Chapter 1

1. Robert L. Phillips, Jr., and Andrew W. Bazemore, "Primary Care and Why It Matters for U.S. Health System Reform," *Health Affairs*, May 2010, 806–810.

2. Institute of Medicine, *Crossing the Quality Chasm: A New Health System for the 21st Century*. Washington, DC: National Academy Press, 2001, 3–4.

3. Elizabeth A. McGlynn, Steven M. Asch, John Adams, Joan Keesey, Jennifer Hicks, Alison DeCristofaro, and Eve A. Kerr, "The Quality of Health Care Delivered to Adults in the United States," *New England Journal of Medicine* 348 (2003): 2635–45.

4. Héctor Bueno, MD, PhD; Joseph S. Ross, MD, MHS; Yun Wang, PhD; Jersey Chen, MD, MPH; María T. Vidán, MD, PhD; Sharon-Lise T. Normand, PhD; Jeptha P. Curtis, MD; Elizabeth E. Drye, MD, SM; Judith H. Lichtman, PhD; Patricia S. Keenan, PhD; Mikhail Kosiborod, MD; and Harlan M. Krumholz, MD, SM, "Trends in Length of Stay and Short-Term Outcomes Among Medicare Patients Hospitalized for Heart Failure, 1993–2006," *JAMA* 303, no. 21 (2010): 2141–2147.

5. Donald M. Berwick, Thomas W. Nolan, and John Whittington, "The Triple Aim: Care, Health and Cost," *Health Affairs*, May/June 2008, 759–769.

6. Gulshan Sharma, MD, MPH; Kathlyn E. Fletcher, MD, MA; Dong Zhang, PhD; Yong-Fang Kuo, PhD; Jean L. Freeman, PhD; and James S. Goodwin, MD, "Continuity of Outpatient and Inpatient Care by Primary Care Physicians for Hospitalized Older Adults," *JAMA* 301, no. 16 (2009): 1671–1680.

7. Karen Davis, PhD; Cathy Schoen, MS; Stephen C. Schoenbaum, MD, MPH; Michelle M. Doty, PhD, MPH; Alyssa L. Holmgren, MPA; Jennifer L. Kriss; and Katherine K. Shea, "Mirror, Mirror on the Wall: An International Update on the Comparative Performance of American Health Care," The Commonwealth Fund, May 15, 2007, accessed at http://www.commonwealthfund.org/Content/Publications/Fund-Reports/2007/May/Mirror—Mirror-on-the-Wall—An-International-Update-on-the-Comparative-Performance-of-American-Healthcare.aspx.

8. Berwick, Nolan, and Whittington, "The Triple Aim" …

9. Ibid.

10. Nicholas Stine, MD, and David Chokshi, MD, "Defining Population Health," Human Capital Blog, RWJ Foundation, Jan. 23, 2013, accessed at http://www.rwjf.org/en/blogs/human-capital-blog/2013/01/defining_population.html

11. David M. Lawrence, "How to Forge a High-Tech Marriage Between Primary Care and Population Health," *Health Affairs*, May 2010, 1004–1009.

12. David M. Lawrence, *From Chaos to Care: The Promise of Team-Based Medicine*(Cambridge, MA: Da Capo Press, 2003).

13. Institute of Medicine, "Crossing the Quality Chasm," 3.

14. Ibid., 181–20.

15. Ken Terry, *Rx for Health Care Reform* (Nashville: Vanderbilt University Press, 2007), 177–178.

16. Patient-Centered Primary Care Collaborative, "Managing Populations, Maximizing Technology: Population Health Management in the Medical Neighborhood," October 2013, accessed at http://www.pcpcc.org/resource/managing-populations-maximizing-technology.

17. SK&A press release, "Small Medical Offices Take Lead in Growth of EHR Adoption, Reveals Exclusive Survey from SK&A," March 24, 2014, accessed at http://www.skainfo.com/press_releases.php?article=122.

18. Meredith B. Rosenthal, Rushika Fernandopulle, HyunSook Ryu Song, and Bruce Landon, "Paying for Quality: Providers' Incentives for Quality Improvement," *Health Affairs*, March/April 2004, 127–141.

19. Thomas Bodenheimer, Edward H. Wagner, and Kevin Grumbach, "Improving Primary Care for Patients with Chronic Illness," *JAMA*288 (2002): 1775–1779.

20. Thomas Bodenheimer, Edward H. Wagner, and Kevin Grumbach, "Improving Primary Care for Patients with Chronic Illness: The Chronic Care Model, Part 2," *JAMA* 288 (2002): 1909–1914.

21. AAFP, AAP, ACP, AOA, "Joint Principles of the Patient-Centered Medical Home," February 2007, accessed at http://www.pcpcc.net/content/joint-principles-patient-centered-medical-home.

22. Paul A. Nutting, MD, MSPH; William L. Miller, MD, MA; Benjamin F. Crabtree, PhD; Carlos Roberto Jaen, MD, PhD; Elizabeth E. Stewart, PhD; and Kurt C. Stange, MD, PhD, "Initial Lessons from the First National Demonstration Project on Practice Transformation to a Patient-Centered Medical Home," *Annals of Family Medicine* 7 (2009): 254–260.

23. Bruce E. Landon, James M. Gill, Richard C. Antonelli, and Eugene C. Rich, "Prospects for Rebuilding Primary Care Using the Patient-Centered Medical Home," *Health Affairs*, May 2010, 827–834.

24. Elliott S. Fisher, Donald M. Berwick, and Karen Davis, "Achieving Healthcare Reform: How Physicians Can Help," *New England Journal of Medicine* 360 (2009): 2495–2497.

25. Diane R. Rittenhouse, Stephen M. Shortell, and Elliott S. Fisher, "Primary Care and Accountable Care—Two Essential Elements of Delivery-System Reform," *New England Journal of Medicine* 361 (2009): 2301–2303.

26. Molly Gamble, "Total Numbers of ACOs Tops 520," *Beckers Hospital Review*, April 24, 2014, accessed at http://www.beckershospitalreview.com/accountable-care-organizations/total-number-of-acos-tops-520.html.

27. Jeff Goldsmith, "The ACO: Not Ready for Prime Time," *Health Affairs Blog*, Aug. 17, 2009, accessed at http://healthaffairs.org/blog/2009/08/17/the-accountable-care-organization-not-ready-for-prime-time/.

28. Lawrence, "How to Forge a High-Tech Marriage" …

29. Ibid.

30. Rushika Fernandopulle and Neil Patel, "How the Electronic Health Record Did Not Measure Up to the Demands of Our Medical Home Practice," *Health Affairs*, April 2010, 622–628.

Chapter 2

1. Kaiser Family Foundation, "Summary of New Health Reform Law," accessed at http://www.kff.org/healthreform/upload/8061.pdf.

2. CMS, "Shared Savings Program," accessed at http://www.cms.gov/Medicare/Medicare-Fee-for-Service-Payment/sharedsavingsprogram/index.html.

3. Blue Shield of California press release, "Blue Shield of California, Catholic Healthcare West & Hill Physicians Medical Group to Pilot Innovative New Care Model for CalPERS," April 22, 2009.

4. Leavitt Partners Center for Accountable Care Intelligence. http://healthaffairs.org/blog/2014/01/29/accountable-care-growth-in-2014-a-look-ahead/.

5. Molly Gamble, "Total Number of ACOs Tops 520," *Beckers Hospital Review*, April 24, 2014, accessed at http://www.beckershospitalreview.com/accountable-care-organizations/total-number-of-acos-tops-520.html.

6. S. Lawrence Kocot, Farzad Mostashari, and Ross White, "Year One Results from Medicare Shared Savings Program: What It Means Going Forward," Brookings Institution Upfront blog, Feb. 7, 2014.

7. Jordan T. Cohen, "A Guide to Accountable Care Organizations, and Their Role in the Senate's Health Reform Bill," *Health Reform Watch*, March 11, 2010, accessed at http://www.healthreformwatch.com/2010/03/11/a-guide-to-accountable-care-organizations-and-their-role-in-the-senates-health-reform-bill/.

8. Ibid.

9. Ken Terry, "Gainsharing Is Becoming More Respectable," *BNET Healthcare*, July 28, 2009, accessed at http://industry.bnet.com/healthcare/1000908/gainsharing-is-becoming-more-respectable/?utm_source=feedburner&utm_medium=feed&utm_ca

mpaign=Feed%3A+bnet%2Fhealthcare+%28BNET+Industr ies+-+Healthcare+Insights%29.

10. Jeff Goldsmith, "The Accountable Care Organization: Not Ready For Prime Time," Health Affairs Blog, August 17, 2009, accessed at http://healthaffairs.org/blog/2009/08/17/the-accountable-care-organization-not-ready-for-prime-time/.

11. Ken Terry, "Physician Alignment," *Hospitals & Health Networks*, September 2009, accessed at http://www.hhnmag.com/hhnmag_app/jsp/articledisplay. jsp?dcrpath=HHNMAG/Article/data/09SEP2009/0909HHN CoverStory_Alignment&domain=HHNMAG.

12. Gregg Blesch, "FTC Offers Clearer Guidance on Clinical Integration Agreements," Modern Physician.com, April 27, 2009, accessed at http:// www.modernphysician.com/apps/pbcs.dll/article?AID=/20090427/ MODERNPHYSICIAN/304199990#.

13. "Online Connectivity: Linking Providers and Patients to Create a Community of Care," *Patient Safety & Quality Healthcare*, January/ February 2010, accessed at http://www.psqh.com/januaryfebruary-2010/391-online-connectivity.html.

14. Ken Terry, "Global Capitation—It's Back," *Physicians Practice*, April 2009, accessed at http://www.physicianspractice.com/index/ fuseaction/articles.details/articleID/1313.htm.

15. Blue Cross Blue Shield of Massachusetts, "Alternative Quality Contract," accessed at http://www.bluecrossma.com/visitor/about-us/ affordability-quality/aqc.html.

16. Blue Shield of California press release, "Blue Shield of California, Catholic Healthcare West & Hill Physicians Medical Group" …

17. Josette N. Gbemudu, Bridget K. Larson, Aricca D. Van Citters, Sara A. Kreindler, Frances M. Wu, Eugene C. Nelson, Stephen M. Shortell, and Elliott S. Fisher, "Healthcare Partners: Building on a Foundation of Global Risk Management to Achieve Accountable Care," Commonwealth Fund case study, January 2012, accessed at http://www.commonwealthfund.org/~/media/Files/Publications/ Case%20Study/2012/Jan/1572_Gbemudu_HealthCare_Partners_ case%20study_01_17_2012.pdf.

18. Brookings-Dartmouth ACO Learning Network, home page at https:// xteam.brookings.edu/bdacoln/Pages/home.aspx.

19. Patient Protection and Affordable Care Act, H.R. 3590, Sec. 3022 (Medicare Shared Savings Program).

20. Berkeley Center on Health, Economic, & Family Security, "Implementing Accountable Care Organizations," Executive Summary, accessed at http://www.law.berkeley.edu/files/chefs/Implementing_ACOs_May_2010.pdf.

21. Gail Wilensky, "Lessons from the Physician Group Practice Demonstration—a Sobering Reflection," *New England Journal of Medicine* 365 (2011): 1659–1661.

22. Harold Dash, MD, "The Everett Clinic's Journey to an Accountable Care Organization," slide presentation, American Medical Group Association Northwest Regional Meeting, June 4, 2010.

23. The Commonwealth Fund, "Mirror, Mirror on the Wall: How The Performance of the U.S. Health Care System Compares Internationally, 2010 Update," accessed at http://www.commonwealthfund.org/Content/Publications/Fund-Reports/2010/Jun/Mirror-Mirror-Update.aspx.

24. Institute of Medicine, *Crossing the Quality Chasm*. Washington, DC: National Academy Press, 2001.

25. David M. Lawrence, "How to Forge a High-Tech Marriage Between Primary Care and Population Health," *Health Affairs*, May 2010, 1004–1009.

26. David M. Lawrence, *From Chaos to Care: The Promise of Team-Based Medicine*. Cambridge, MA: Da Capo Press, 2003.

27. AAFP, AAP, ACP, AOA, "Joint Principles of the Patient-Centered Medical Home," February 2007, accessed at http://www.pcpcc.net/content/joint-principles-patient-centered-medical-home.

28. Paul A. Nutting, MD, MSPH; William L. Miller, MD, MA; Benjamin F. Crabtree, PhD; Carlos Roberto Jaen, MD, PhD; Elizabeth E. Stewart, PhD; and Kurt C. Stange, MD, PhD, "Initial Lessons from the First National Demonstration Project on Practice Transformation to a Patient-Centered Medical Home," *Annals of Family Medicine* 7 (2009): 254–260.

29. Greg Slabodkin, "HIE Among Hospitals Grows, Still Needs Improvement," *Health Data Management*, May 6, 2014, accessed at http://www.healthdatamanagement.com/news/HIE-Among-Hospitals-

Needs-Improvement-47997-1.html?utm_campaign=daily-may%
206%202014&utm_medium=email&utm_source=newsletter&ET=
healthdatamanagement%3Ae2629612%3A3696614a%3A&st=email.

30. Julia Adler-Milstein, David W. Bates, and Ashish K. Jha, "Operational Health Information Exchanges Show Substantial Growth, But Long-Term Funding Remains a Concern," *Health Affairs* 32, no. 8 (August 2013): 1486–1492.

31. Ken Terry, "KLAS: 'Private' HIEs Leaving 'Public' HIEs in the Dust," FierceHealthIT, July 8, 2011, accessed at http://www.fiercehealthit. com/story/klas-private-hies-leaving-public-hies-dust/2011-07-08.

32. HIT Trends blog, April 2014, accessed at http://www.directtrust.org/ storage/post-images/HIT%20Trends%20April%202014.pdf.

33. Rushika Fernandopulle and Neil Patel, "How the Electronic Health Record Did Not Measure Up to the Demands of Our Medical Home Practice," *Health Affairs*, April 2010, 622–628.

Chapter 3

1. Madeline Hyden, "70 Percent of Study Participants Moving Toward PCMH Model, MGMA Research Reveals," MGMA blog post, July 20, 2011.

2. NCQA, "The Future of Patient-Centered Medical Homes," accessed at http://www.ncqa.org/Portals/0/Public%20Policy/2014%20Comment %20Letters/The_Future_of_PCMH.pdf.

3. NCQA, "Formal NCQA PCMH Sponsoring Organizations," accessed at http://www.ncqa.org/Portals/0/Programs/Recognition/PCMH/ Compiled_List_3_1_2014.pdf.

4. NCQA, "Payers Using Recognition," accessed at http://www.ncqa.org/ tabid/131/Default.aspx.

5. Patient Centered Primary Care Collaborative, "Benefits of Implementing the Primary Care Patient-Centered Medical Home: A Review of Cost & Quality Results, 2012," accessed at http://www.pcpcc.org/sites/default/ files/media/benefits_of_implementing_the_primary_care_pcmh.pdf.

6. Centers for Medicare and Medicaid, "Multi-payer Primary Care Practice Demonstration Fact Sheet," accessed at http://www.cms.

gov/Medicare/Demonstration-Projects/DemoProjectsEvalRpts/
downloads/mapcpdemo_Factsheet.pdf.

7. Patient Centered Primary Care Collaborative, "Benefits of Implementing the"…

8. Sarah Klein, "The Veterans Health Administration: Implementing Patient-Centered Medical Homes in the Nation's Largest Integrated Delivery System," The Commonwealth Fund, September 13, 2011, accessed at http://www.commonwealthfund.org/publications/case-studies/2011/sep/va-medical-homes

9. PCPCC, "Evidence of the Effectiveness of PCMH on Quality of Care and Cost," accessed at http://www.amsa.org/AMSA/Libraries/Committee_Docs/Evidence_Supporting_the_PCMH_Model.sflb.ashx

10. Kevin Grumbach, Thomas Bodenheimer, and Paul Grundy, "The Outcomes of Implementing Patient-Centered Medical Home Demonstrations: A Review of the Evidence on Quality, Access and Costs from Recent Prospective Evaluation Studies," August 2009, paper prepared for PCPCC.

11. Ibid.

12. Paul A. Nutting, Benjamin J. Crabtree, William L. Miller, Kurt C. Stange, Elizabeth Stewart, and Carlos Jaen, "Transforming Physician Practices to Patient-Centered Medical Homes: Lessons from the National Demonstration Project," *Health Affairs* 30, no. 3 (March 2011): 439–445.

13. Marci Nielsen, CEO, PCPCC, "Show Me the Data: Do Patient-Centered Medical Homes Work?" presentation, June 9, 2014.

14. Paul Grundy, Kay R. Hagan, Jennie Chin Hansen, and Kevin Grumbach, "The Multi-Stakeholder Movement for Primary Care Renewal and Reform," *Health Affairs* 29, no. 5 (2010): 791–798.

15. Ibid.

16. Ibid.

17. Suzanna Felt-Lisk and Tricia Higgins, "Exploring the Promise of Population Health Management Programs to Improve Health," Mathematica Policy Research Issue Brief, August 2011, accessed at http://www.mathematica-mpr.com/publications/pdfs/health/PHM_brief.pdf.

18. David Nash, "Healthcare Reform's Rx for Primary Care," *MedPage Today*, Aug. 18, 2010, accessed at http://www.medpagetoday.com/Columns/21750.

19. American Academy of Family Practice, American Academy of Pediatrics, American College of Physicians, and American Osteopathic Association, "Joint Principles of the Patient-Centered Medical Home," March 2007, accessed at http://www.acponline.org/running_practice/delivery_and_payment_models/pcmh/demonstrations/jointprinc_05_17.pdf

20. Bruce E. Landon, James M. Gill, Richard C. Antonelli, and Eugene C. Rich, "Prospects for Rebuilding Primary Care Using the Patient-Centered Medical Home," *Health Affairs* 29, no. 5 (2010): 827–834.

21. Blue Cross and Blue Shield Association, slide presentation, "The Patient-Centered Medical Home: BC/BS Pilot Initiatives," slides 22 and 24.

22. NCQA, "Physician Practice Connections," accessed at http://www.ncqa.org/Default.aspx?tabid=141.

23. NCQA, "Physician Practice Connections—Patient-Centered Medical Home," accessed at http://www.ncqa.org/tabid/631/Default.aspx.

24. Margaret E. O'Kane and Patricia Barrett, "Sneak Preview: 2014 Patient-Centered Medical Home Recognition," NCQA slides, March 10, 2014, accessed at https://www.ncqa.org/Portals/0/Newsroom/2014/PCMH%202014%20Press%20Preview%20FINAL%20Slides.pdf.

25. Ken Terry, "Medical Specialists Encouraged to Use More IT," *InformationWeek Healthcare*, June 13, 2012, accessed at http://www.informationweek.com/healthcare/policy/medical-specialists-encouraged-to-use-mo/240001986.

26. US Agency for Healthcare Research and Quality, "Practice-Based Population Health: Information Technology to Support Transformation to Proactive Primary Care," July 2010, accessed at http://pcmh.ahrq.gov/sites/default/files/attachments/Information%20Technology%20to%20Support%20Transformation%20to%20Proactive%20Primary%20Care.pdf

27. Diane R. Rittenhouse, Lawrence P. Casalino, Robin R. Gillies, Stephen M. Shortell, and Bernard Lau, "Measuring the Medical Home: Infrastructure in Large Groups," *Health Affairs* 27, no. 5 (2008): 1246–1258.

28. Diane R. Rittenhouse, Lawrence P. Casalino, Stephen M. Shortell, Sean R. McClellan, Robin R. Gillies, Jeffrey A. Alexander, and Melinda L. Drum, "Small and Medium-Sized Physician Practices Use Few Patient-Centered Medical Home Processes," *Health Affairs* 30, no. 8 (2012): 1575–1584.

29. Paul A. Nutting, MD, MSPH; William L. Miller, MD, MA; Benjamin F. Crabtree, PhD; Carlos Roberto Jaen, MD, PhD; Elizabeth E. Stewart, PhD; and Kurt C. Stange, MD, PhD, "Initial Lessons from the First National Demonstration Project on Practice Transformation to a Patient-Centered Medical Home," *Annals of Family Medicine* 7 (2009): 254–260.

30. Landon, Gill, Antonelli, and Rich, "Prospects for Rebuilding Primary Care" …

31. Ibid.

32. Phytel press release, "VHA, TransforMED and Phytel Awarded $20.75 Million Health Care Innovation Grant," June 20, 2012.

33. Katie Merrell and Robert A. Berenson, "Structured Payment for Medical Homes," *Health Affairs* 29, no. 5 (2010): 852–858.

34. Grundy, Hagan, Hansen, and Grumbach, "The Multi-Stakeholder Movement for" …

35. Blue Cross and Blue Shield Association, "The Patient-Centered Medical Home" …, slide 25.

36. Robert A. Berenson, "Payment Approaches and Cost of the Patient-Centered Medical Home," presentation at PCPCC meeting, July 16, 2008, slide 25.

37. Robert S. Nocon, Ravi Sharma, Jonathan M. Birnberg, Quyen Ngo-Metzger, Sang Mee Lee, and Marshall H. Chin, "Association Between Patient-Centered Medical Home Rating and Operating Cost at Federally Funded Health Centers," *JAMA* 308, no. 1 (2012): 60–66.

38. US Agency for Healthcare Research and Quality, "Practice-Based Population Health" …

39. Nutting, Miller, Crabtree, Jaen, Stewart, and Stange, "Initial Lessons from the First National Demonstration Project" …

40. US Agency for Healthcare Research and Quality, "Practice-Based Population Health" …

41. Ken Terry, "Do Disease Registries=$$rewards?" *Medical Economics*, Nov. 4, 2005, accessed at http://medicaleconomics.modernmedicine.com/memag/article/articleDetail.jsp?id=190114&pageID=1&sk=&date=.

42. Neil Versel, "Reimbursement for Home Monitoring Gradually Expands," Mobihealth News, Sept. 26, 2013, accessed at http://mobihealthnews.com/25823/reimbursement-for-home-monitoring-gradually-expands/

Chapter 4

1. Department of Health and Human Services press release, "Doctors' and hospitals' use of health IT more than doubles since 2012," May 22, 2013, accessed at http://www.hhs.gov/news/press/2013pres/05/20130522a.html.

2. Kaiser Family Foundation, "Summary of the Affordable Care Act," accessed at http://kaiserfamilyfoundation.files.wordpress.com/2011/04/8061-021.pdf.

3. Centers for Medicare and Medicaid Services, "Multi-payer Primary Care Practice Demonstration Fact Sheet," accessed at http://www.cms.gov/Medicare/Demonstration-Projects/DemoProjectsEvalRpts/downloads/mapcpdemo_Factsheet.pdf.

4. Centers for Disease Control and Prevention, "Meaningful Use," accessed at http://www.cdc.gov/ehrmeaningfuluse/introduction.html.

5. CMS, "Medicare and Medicaid Health Information Technology: Title IV of the American Recovery and Reinvestment Act," fact sheet, June 16, 2009, accessed at https://www.cms.gov/apps/me0dia/press/factsheet.asp?Counter=3466&intNumPerPage=10&checkDate=&checkKey=&srchType=1&numDays=3500&srchOpt=0&srchData=&keywordType=All&chkNewsType=6&intPage=&showAll=&pYear=&year=&desc=&cboOrder=date.

6. HHS (Department of Health and Human Services)/CMS, "Medicare and Medicaid Programs; Electronic Health Record Program; Final Rule," Federal Register, 42 CFR Parts 412, 413, 422, and 495.

7. HHS (Department of Health and Human Services)/CMS, "Medicare and Medicaid Programs; Electronic Health Record Program; Proposed

Rule," aka "Notice of Proposed Rulemaking," Federal Register, 42 CFR Parts 412, 413, 422. and 495: 1852.

8. CMS, "Medicare and Medicaid EHR Incentive Program Basics," accessed at http://www.cms.gov/Regulations-and-Guidance/Legislation/EHR IncentivePrograms/Basics.html.

9. Ibid.

10. CMS, "An Introduction to Medicaid EHR Incentive Program for Eligible Professionals," accessed at http://www.cms.gov/Regulations-and-Guidance/Legislation/EHRIncentivePrograms/Downloads/EHR_Medicaid_BegGuide_Stage1.pdf.

11. Ken Terry, "Feds Extend Deadline for Electronic Health Meaningful Use," *InformationWeek Healthcare,*" Dec. 9, 2013, accessed at http://www.informationweek.com/healthcare/policy-and-regulation/feds-extend-deadline-for-electronic-health-meaningful-use—-/d/d-id/1112990.

12. CMS, "Medicare and Medicaid EHR Incentive Program Basics" …

13. CMS press release, "CMS Rule to Help Providers Make Use of Certified EHR Technology," May 20, 2014, accessed at http://www.cms.gov/Newsroom/MediaReleaseDatabase/Press-releases/2014-Press-releases-items/2014-05-20.html.

14. CMS, "An Introduction to Medicare EHR Incentive Program for Eligible Professionals," accessed at http://www.cms.gov/Regulations-and-Guidance/Legislation/EHRIncentivePrograms/Downloads/EHR_Medicare_Stg1_BegGuide.pdf.

15. HHS (Department of Health and Human Services)/CMS, "Medicare and Medicaid Programs; Electronic Health Record Program; Final Rule," Federal Register, 42 CFR Parts 412, 413, 422, and 495.

16. CMS press release, "CMS Rule to Help Providers" …

17. CSC, "Summary of Key Provisions in Final Rule for Stage 2 HITECH Meaningful Use," Nov. 28, 2012, accessed at http://assets1.csc.com/health_services/downloads/CSC_Key_Provisions_of_Final_Rule_for_Stage_2.pdf.

18. Ibid.

19. Terry, "CMS Reminds Physicians of Meaningful Use Hardship Exception Deadline," *Medscape Medical News*, May 8, 2014, accessed at http://www.medscape.com/viewarticle/824823.

20. iHealthBeat, "Review of Q1 Federal Health IT Activity," April 21, 2014, accessed at http://www.ihealthbeat.org/insight/2014/review-of-q1-2014-federal-health-it-activity.

21. Health IT Policy Committee, Meaningful Use Workgroup, "Stage 3 Draft Recommendations," March 11, 2014, accessed at http://www.healthit.gov/FACAS/sites/faca/files/HITPC_MUWG_Stage3_Recs_2014-03-11_v6_0.pdf.

22. Ibid.

23. CMS, "Stage 2 Eligible Professional Meaningful Use Core and Menu Measures," October 2012, accessed at http://www.cms.gov/Regulations-and-Guidance/Legislation/EHRIncentivePrograms/Downloads/Stage2_MeaningfulUseSpecSheet_TableContents_EPs.pdf.

24. Terry, "KLAS: 'Private' HIEs Leaving 'Public' HIEs in the Dust," FierceHealthIT, July 8, 2011, accessed at http://www.fiercehealthit.com/story/klas-private-hies-leaving-public-hies-dust/2011-07-08.

25. Greg Slabodkin, "HIE Among Hospitals Grows, Still Needs Improvement," *Health Data Management*, May 6, 2014, accessed at http://www.healthdatamanagement.com/news/HIE-Among-Hospitals-Needs-Improvement-47997-1.html.

26. ONC, "Dr. Ted Wymyslo Discusses How Health Information Exchange Supports Meaningful Use," accessed at http://www.healthit.gov/providers-professionals/dr-ted-wymyslo-discusses-how-health-information-exchange-supports-meaningful.

27. DirectTrust home page, http://www.directtrust.org.

28. HIMSS, "HIE and Meaningful Use Stage 2 Matrix," accessed at http://www.himss.org/files/HIMSSorg/content/files/MU2_HIE_Matrix_FINAL.pdf.

29. Mary Jo Deering, "ONC Issue Brief: Patient-Generated Health Data and Health IT," Dec. 20, 2013, accessed at http://www.healthit.gov/buzz-blog/electronic-health-and-medical-records/advancing-patient-generated-information-improve-health-care/

30. Ibid.

31. William Van Doomik, "Meaningful Use of Patient-Generated Data in EHRs," blog of American Health Information Management Association, accessed at http://library.ahima.org/xpedio/groups/public/documents/ahima/bok1_050394.hcsp?dDocName=bok1_050394.

32. iHealthBeat, "Concern Grows About Doctor Offices Opting Out of Meaningful Use," Dec. 23, 2013, accessed at http://www.ihealthbeat.org/articles/2013/12/23/concern-grows-about-doctor-offices-opting-out-of-meaningful-use.

33. Mark Hagland, "Dr. Halamka's Dramatic MU Prediction in Boston," *Healthcare Informatics*, May 13, 2014, accessed at http://www.healthcare-informatics.com/blogs/mark-hagland/dr-halamka-s-dramatic-mu-prediction-boston.

Chapter 5

1. Eugene Kroch, R. Wesley Champion, Susan D. DeVore, Marla R. Kugel, Danielle A. Lloyd, and Lynne Rothney-Kozlak, "Measuring Progress Toward Accountable Care," 19, Premier Research Institute, Dec. 2012.

2. Wayne J. Guglielmo, "The Feds Ease Antitrust Rules—Cautiously," *Medical Economics*, June 21, 2002, accessed at http://medical economics.modernmedicine.com/medical-economics/news/feds-ease-antitrust-rules-cautiously?page=full.

3. Alicia Gallegos, "Clinical Integration Model Gets FTC Green Light," *AM News*, March 11, 2013, accessed at http://www.amednews.com/article/20130311/government/130319976/6/.

4. James J. Pizzo and Mark E. Grube, "Getting to There From Here: Evolving to ACOs Through Clinical Integration Programs, Including the Advocate Health Care Example as Presented by Lee B. Sacks, M.D.," Kaufman, Hall & Associates, 2011, accessed at http://www.advocatehealth.com/documents/app/ci_to_aco.pdf.

5. Premier Healthcare Alliance, presentation, "Clinically Integrated Networks: a Population Health Building Block," 2013.

6. Kroch, Champion, DeVore, Kugel, Lloyd, and Rothney-Kozlak, "Measuring Progress Toward Accountable Care," 6.

7. Institute for Health Technology Transformation, "Population Health Management: A Roadmap for Provider-Based Automation in a New Era of Healthcare," 2012, accessed at http://ihealthtran.com/pdf/PHMReport.pdf.

8. Ibid.

9. Ashok Rai, Paul Prichard, Richard Hodach, and Ted Courtemanche, "Using Physician-Led Automated Communications to Improve Patient Health," *Journal of Population Health Management*, Vol. 14, 00, 2011. doi:10.1089/pop.2010.0033.

10. Centers for Medicare and Medicaid Services, "Stage 1 vs. Stage 2 Comparison Table for Eligible Professionals," August 2012, accessed at https://www.cms.gov/Regulations-and-Guidance/Legislation/EHRIncentivePrograms/Downloads/Stage1vsStage2CompTablesforEP.pdf.

11. Ann-Lisa Silvestre, Valerie M. Sue, and Jill Y. Allen, "If You Build It, Will They Come? The Kaiser Permanente Model of Online Healthcare," *Health Affairs* 28, no. 2 (2009): 334–344.

12. Sarah O'Hara, "Next-Generation Clinical Integration: Early Findings from a New Research Initiative," Network Advantage blog, The Advisory Board Co., Jan. 30, 2012, accessed at http://www.advisory.com/Research/Health-Care-Advisory-Board/Blogs/Network-Advantage/2012/01/Next-generation-clinical-integration-early-findings-from-a-new-research-initiative.

13. Mark C. Shields, Pankaj H. Patel, Martin Manning, and Lee Sacks, "A Model for Integrating Independent Physicians into Accountable Care Organizations," *Health Affairs* 30, no. 1 (2011): 161–172.

14. Annie Lowrey, "A Health Provider Strives to Keep Hospital Beds Empty," *New York Times*, April 23, 2013.

Chapter 6

1. Marc L. Berk and Alan C. Monheit, "The Concentration of Health Care Expenditures, Revisited," *Health Affairs* 20, no. 2 (March/April 2001).

2. Agency for Healthcare Research and Quality, "The High Concentration of U.S. Health Care Expenditures," *Research in Action*, Issue 19, June 2006.

3. HIMSS Analytics, "Clinical Analytics in the World of Meaningful Use," Feb. 2011, accessed at http://www.himss.org/content/files/20110221_Anvita.pdf.

4. HIMSS Analytics, "Clinical Analytics: Can Organizations Maximize Clinical Data?" June 7, 2010, accessed at http://www.himss.org/content/files/Clinical_Analytics.pdf.

5. E. Ben-Chetri, C. Chen-Shuali, E. Zimran, G. Munter, and G. Nesher, "A Simplified Scoring Tool for Prediction of Readmission in Elderly Patients Hospitalized in Internal Medicine Departments," *Israeli Medical Association Journal*, 14, no. 12 (Dec. 2012): 752–6.

6. J. Donze, D. Aujesky, D. Williams, and J. L. Schnipper, "Potentially Avoidable 30-Day Hospital Readmissions in Medical Patients: Derivation and Validation of a Prediction Model," *JAMA Internal Medicine* 173, no. 8 (Apr. 22, 2013): 632–8, doi:10.1001/jamainternmed.2013.3023.

7. Ken Terry, "Futuristic Clinical Decision Support Tool Catches On," *InformationWeek Healthcare*, Jan. 27, 2012, accessed at http://www.informationweek.com/healthcare/clinical-systems/futuristic-clinical-decision-support-too/232500603.

8. J. Frank Wharam and Jonathan P. Weiner, "The Promise and Peril of Healthcare Forecasting," *American Journal of Managed Care* 18, no. 3 (2012):e82–e85), 2.

9. Centers for Disease Control and Prevention, "The Power to Prevent, the Call to Control: At a Glance 2009," accessed at http://www.cdc.gov/chronicdisease/resources/publications/aag/chronic.htm.

10. James D. Reschovsky, Jack Hadley, and Ellyn R. Boukus, "Following the Money: Factors Associated with the Cost of Treating High-Cost Medicare Beneficiaries," *Health Services Research Journal* 46, no. 4 (Aug. 2011): 997–1021. Accessed at http://www.ncbi.nlm.nih.gov/pmc/articles/PMC3165175/.

11. Terry, "ACOs Need Claims Data for Analytics, Expert Says," *InformationWeek Healthcare*, Sept. 16, 2013, accessed at http://www.informationweek.com/healthcare/electronic-medical-records/acos-need-claims-data-for-analytics-expe/240161353.

12. Colorado Beacon Consortium, Issue Brief, Vol. 2, Issue 2, accessed at http://origin.library.constantcontact.com/download/get/file/1101292888704-1346/CBC-v2%232.edits2.pdf.

13. Ian Duncan, *Healthcare Risk Adjustment and Predictive Modeling* (Winstead, CT: ACTEX Publications, 2011).

14. Centers for Medicare and Medicaid Services, "Chronic Conditions Among Medicare Beneficiaries: 2012 Chartbook," accessed at http://www.cms.gov/Research-Statistics-Data-and-Systems/Statistics-Trends-and-Reports/Chronic-Conditions/Downloads/2012Chartbook.pdf.

15. Colorado Beacon Consortium, Issue Brief, Vol. 2, Issue 2 …, p. 2.

16. Johns Hopkins University, "The Johns Hopkins ACG System: Performance Assessment," accessed at http://acg.jhsph.org/index.php?option=com_content&view=article&id=88&Itemid=116.

17. Personal communication with Ron Russell, Verisk.

18. Colorado Beacon Consortium, Issue Brief, Vol. 2, Issue 2 …

19. Terry, "ACOs Need Claims Data for Analytics" …

20. HIMSS Analytics, "Clinical Analytics in the World of Meaningful Use" …

21. Institute for Health Technology Transformation, "Analytics: The Nervous System of IT-Enabled Healthcare," 2013, accessed at http://ihealthtran.com/iHT2analyticsreport.pdf?utm_source=hubspot_automated_email&utm_medium=email&utm_content=8621800&_hsenc=p2ANqtz_AX0J4DkSaUDYHHQOvx k2VkqyV9taFucUh4JoeGzcz4x2AANUTXSLKUg1TIrDTBNNY dU7RN4EkDkAeqXrdG5dM4Q9ElQ&_hsmi=8621800.

22. Ian MacDowell, *Measuring Health: A Guide to Rating Scales and Questionnaires, Third Edition* (Oxford: Oxford University Press, 2006), accessed at http://a4ebm.org/sites/default/files/Measuring%20Health.pdf.

23. Office of the National Coordinator for Health IT, Factsheet, Greater Cincinnati Beacon Collaboration (Cincinnati, OH).

Chapter 7

1. Beth Kutscher, "Hospitals on the Rebound, Showing Stronger Operating Margins," *Modern Healthcare*, Jan. 3, 2014, accessed at http://www.modernhealthcare.com/article/20140103/NEWS/301039973.

2. Jenna Levy, "U.S. Uninsured Rate Drops So Far in First Quarter of 2014," Gallup Well-Being, Feb. 12, 2014, accessed at http://www.gallup.com/poll/167393/uninsured-rate-drops-far-first-quarter-2014.aspx?utm_source=H2RMinutes+HIX+Feb.+20%2C+2014&utm_campaign=HIX+Minutes+2%2F20%2F14&utm_medium=email.

3. Kaiser Family Foundation, "Status of State Action on the Medicaid Expansion Decision, 2014," accessed at http://kff.org/health-reform/state-indicator/state-activity-around-expanding-medicaid-under-the-affordable-care-act/.

4. MSN Money, "High Deductibles Fuel New Worries of Obamacare Sticker Shock," Dec. 9, 2013, accessed at http://money.msn.com/health-and-life-insurance/article.aspx?post=0ad0d4e9-221f-4df8-9239-ac92ee6b222b.

5. Lindsey Dunn, "Narrow Networks Put Hospitals on the Offensive," *Becker's Hospital Review,* Jan. 31, 2014, accessed at http://www.beckershospitalreview.com/healthcare-blog/narrow-networks-put-hospitals-on-the-offensive.html.

6. American Hospital Association, "Underpayment by Medicare and Medicaid Fact Sheet, 2014," accessed at http://www.aha.org/content/14/2012-medicare-med-underpay.pdf.

7. AHA, "Uncompensated Hospital Care Cost Fact Sheet," January 2014, accessed at http://www.aha.org/content/14/14uncompensatedcare.pdf.

8. Leemore Dafny, "Hospital Industry Consolidation—Still More to Come?" *New England Journal of Medicine* 370 (2014): 198–199.

9. Aubrey Westgate, "Getting Paid for Value: Defining New Reimbursement Models," *Physicians Practice,* Jan. 27, 2014, accessed at http://www.physicianspractice.com/fee-schedule-survey/getting-paid-value-defining-new-reimbursement-models?GUID=03976E2A-4C81-4F0B-BC95-41358DBB7419&rememberme=1&ts=31012014.

10. William E. Encinosa and Jaeyong Bae, "Will Meaningful Use Electronic Medical Records Reduce Hospital Costs?" *American Journal of Managed Care* 19 (11) spec. no. 10 (Nov. 22, 2013): eS19–eSP25, accessed at http://www.ajmc.com/publications/issue/2013/2013-11-vol19-sp/Will-Meaningful-Use-Electronic-Medical-Records-Reduce-Hospital-Costs.

11. American Medical Association, letter to Department of Health and Human Services, Feb. 12, 2014, accessed at http://www.ama-assn.org/resources/doc/washington/icd-10-letter-to-cms-12feb2014.pdf.

12. AHA, "Payment Cuts to Hospitals Since 2010," accessed at http://www.aha.org/content/14/cumulative-cuts.pdf.

13. Centers for Medicare and Medicaid Services, "Readmissions Reduction Program," accessed at http://www.cms.gov/Medicare/Medicare-Fee-for-Service-Payment/AcuteInpatientPPS/Readmissions-Reduction-Program.html.

14. Maureen McKinney, "Medicare Payments Cut for More Than 1,400 Hospitals Under Value-Based Purchasing Program," *Modern Healthcare*, Nov. 15, 2013, accessed at http://www.modernhealthcare.com/article/20131115/NEWS/311159950.

15. CMS, "Summary of 2015 Physician Value-Based Payment Modifier Policies," accessed at https://www.cms.gov/Medicare/Medicare-Fee-for-Service-Payment/PhysicianFeedbackProgram/Downloads/CY2015ValueModifierPolicies.pdf.

16. Ken Terry, "Pay for Performance Doesn't Make Docs Jump and Shout," CBS Money Watch, March 11, 2009, accessed at http://www.cbsnews.com/news/pay-for-performance-doesnt-make-docs-jump-and-shout/.

17. NCQA slide presentation, "Sneak Preview: 2014 Patient-Centered Medical Home Recognition," March 10, 2014, accessed at https://www.ncqa.org/Portals/0/Newsroom/2014/PCMH%202014%20Press%20Preview%20FINAL%20Slides.pdf.

18. Leavitt Partners, "Growth and Dispersion of Accountable Care Organizations," August 2013 update, accessed at http://leavittpartners.com/wp-content/uploads/2013/11/Growth-and-Disperson-of-ACOs-August-2013.pdf.

19. Decision Resources Group, "Healthcare Reform Continues to Roil U.S. Managed Markets as the Number of ACOs Nearly Doubles and State Exchanges Create Clear Winners and Losers," press release, Feb. 27, 2014, accessed at https://decisionresourcesgroup.com/News-and-Events/Press-Releases/Sift-Through-the-Noise-Healthcare-Reform-022714.

20. American College of Physicians, "Detailed Summary—Medicare Shared Savings/Accountable Care Organization (ACO) Program,"

accessed at http://www.acponline.org/running_practice/delivery_ and_payment_models/aco/aco_detailed_sum.pdf.

21. Ken Terry, "Why Are Insurers Buying Physician Groups?" Hospitals and Health Networks, Jan. 1, 2012, accessed at http://www.hhnmag. com/display/HHN-news-article.dhtml?dcrPath=/templatedata/ HF Common/NewsArticle/data/HHN/Magazine/2012/ Jan/0112HHN_FEA_trendwatching.

22. ACP detailed summary.

23. CMS, "Bundled Payments for Care Improvement (BPCI) Initiative: General Information," accessed at http://innovation.cms.gov/initiatives/ bundled-payments/.

24. Institute for Health Technology Transformation, "Episode Analytics: Essential Tools for New Healthcare Models," accessed at http://www. ihealthtran.com/episode_analytics.html.

25. Julia Adler-Milstein, "A Survey Analysis Suggests That Electronic Health Records Will Yield Revenue Gains for Some Practices and Losses for Many," *Health Affairs* 32, no. 3 (March 2013): 562–570, accessed at http://content.healthaffairs.org/content/32/3/562.abstract.

26. Robert H. Miller, Christopher West, Tiffany Martin Brown, Ida Sim, and Chris Ganchoff, "The Value of Electronic Health Records in Solo or Small Group Practices," *Health Affairs* 24, no. 5 (Sept 2005): 1127–1137, accessed at http://content.healthaffairs.org/content/24/5/1127.abstract.

27. C. M. Cusack, A. D. Knudsen, J. L. Kronstadt, R. F. Singer, and A. L. Brown, "Practice-Based Population Health: Information Technology to Support Transformation to Proactive Primary Care," Agency for Healthcare Research and Quality, July 2010.

28. HIMSS press release, "HIMSS Introduces Health IT Value Suite to Realize the Value of Health IT," July 16, 2013, accessed at http://www. himss.org/News/NewsDetail.aspx?ItemNumber=21536.

29. Care Continuum Alliance, "Advancing the Population Health Improvement Model," http://www.fiercehealthit.com/story/hennepin- health-project-looks-build-countywide-ehr-program-national- implica/2012-01-10.

30. Mitesh S. Patel, Martin J. Arron, Thomas A. Sinsky, Eric H. Green, David W. Baker, Judith L. Bowen, and Susan Day, "Estimating the Staffing Infrastructure for a Patient-Centered Medical Home," *American*

Journal of Managed Care 1, no. 19 (June 21, 2013): N6, accessed at http://www.ajmc.com/publications/issue/2013/2013-1-vol19-n6/estimating-the-staffing-infrastructure-for-a-patient-centered-medical-home/1.

31. Patient-Centered Primary Care Collaborative, "The Patient-Centered Medical Home: An Annual Update of the Evidence, 2012-2013," January 2014, accessed at http://www.pcpcc.org/sites/default/files/resources/4%20-%20Executive%20Summary%20and%20Evidence.pdf.

32. Department of Health and Human Services press release, "Medicare's Delivery System Reform Initiatives Achieve Significant Savings and Quality Improvements—Off to a Strong Start," Jan. 30, 2014, accessed at http://www.hhs.gov/news/press/2014pres/01/20140130a.html.

33. Ashok Rai, Paul Prichard, Richard Hodach, and Ted Courtemanche, "Using Physician-Led Automated Communications to Improve Patient Health," *Population Health Management* 14, no. 4 (Aug. 2011): 175–180.

34. VHA press release, "VHA, TransforMED and Phytel Awarded $20.75 Million Health Care Innovation Challenge Grant," June 20, 2012, accessed at https://www.vha.com/AboutVHA/PressRoom/PressReleases/Pages/VHATransforMEDPhytelChallengegrant.aspx.

35. CMS Readmissions Reduction Program, fact sheet, accessed at http://www.cms.gov/Medicare/Medicare-Fee-for-Service-Payment/AcuteInpatientPPS/Readmissions-Reduction-Program.html.

36. CMS, HCAHPS fact sheet, accessed at http://www.hcahpsonline.org/files/HCAHPS%20Fact%20Sheet%20May%202012.pdf.

37. Jordan Rau, "Methodology: How Value Based Purchasing Payments Are Calculated," Kaiser Health News, Nov. 14, 2013, accessed at http://www.kaiserhealthnews.org/stories/2013/november/14/value-based-purchasing-medicare-methodology.aspx.

Chapter 8

1. Karen Davis, Cathy Schoen, and Kristof Stremikis, "Mirror, Mirror on the Wall: How the Performance of the U.S. Health Care System Compares Internationally, 2010 Update," report of the Commonwealth Fund, June 23, 2010, accessed at http://www.commonwealthfund.org/Publications/Fund-Reports/2010/Jun/Mirror-Mirror-Update.aspx.

2. The Commonwealth Fund, Dartmouth Institute for Clinical Policy and Practice, and Patient Centered Primary Care Collaborative, "Better to Best: Value-Driving Elements of the Patient Centered Medical Home and Accountable Care Organizations," March 2011, 8, accessed at http://www.pcpcc.org/sites/default/files/media/better_best_guide_full_2011.pdf.

3. L. Casalino, R. R. Gillies, S. M. Shortell, J. A. Schmittdiel, T. Bodenheimer, J. C. Robinson, T. Rundall, N. Oswald, H. Schauffler, and M. C. Wang, "External Incentives, Information Technology, and Organized Processes to Improve Health Care Quality for Patients with Chronic Diseases," *JAMA* 289, no. 4 (Jan. 22–29, 2003): 434–41.

4. Patient-Centered Primary Care Collaborative webinar, "Focusing Care Coordination," Mary Kay Owens.

5. Ann S. O'Malley and Peter J. Cunningham, "Patient Experiences with Coordination of Care: The Benefit of Continuity and Primary Care Physician as Referral Source," *Journal of General Internal Medicine* 24, no. 2, 170–177.

6. Emily Carrier, Tracy Yee, and Rachel A. Holzwart, "Coordination Between Emergency and Primary Care Physicians," NIHCR Research Brief No. 3, Feb. 2011, accessed at http://www.nihcr.org/ED-Coordination.html.

7. Hoangmai H. Pham, Joy M. Grossman, Genna R. Cohen, and Thomas Bodenheimer, "Hospitalists and Care Transitions: The Divorce of Inpatient and Outpatient Care," *Health Affairs* 27, no. 5 (Sept./Oct. 2008): 1315–1327.

8. Ann S. O'Malley and James D. Reschovsky, "Referral and Consultation Communication Between Primary Care Doctors and Specialist Physicians: Finding Common Ground," *Archives of Internal Medicine* 171, no. 1.

9. Michael Trisolini, Jyoti Aggarwal, Musetta Leung, Gregory Pope, and John Kautter, "The Medicare Physician Group Practice Demonstration: Lessons Learned on Improving Quality and Efficiency in Health Care," *Commonwealth Fund*, February 2008, 40.

10. Richard J. Baron and Emily Desnouee, "The Struggle to Support Patients' Effort to Change Their Unhealthy Behavior," *Health Affairs* 29 (May 2010): 953–955.

11. O'Malley, "Tapping the Unmet Potential of Health Information Technology," *New England Journal of Medicine*, March 23, 2011.

12. Daniel Fields, Elizabeth Leshen, and Kevita Patel, "Driving Quality Gains and Cost Savings Through Adoption of Medical Homes," *Health Affairs* 29 (May 2010): 819–826.

13. O'Malley, "Tapping the Unmet Potential of Health Information Technology" ...

14. AHRQ, "Closing the Quality Gap: A Critical Analysis of Quality Improvement Strategies," Chapter 7—Care Coordination.

15. Ibid.

16. CMS fact sheet, Medicare Physician Group Practice Demonstration, December 2010, accessed at http://www.cms.gov/DemoProjectsEvalRpts/downloads/PGP_Fact_Sheet.pdf.

17. CMS press release, "Physician Group Practice Demonstration Succeeded in Improving Quality and Reducing Costs," Aug. 8, 2011, accessed at http://www.cms.gov/Medicare/Demonstration-Projects/DemoProjectsEvalRpts/Downloads/PGP_PR.pdf.

18. CMS, "Evaluation of the Medicare Physician Group Practice Demonstration," September 2012, accessed at http://www.cms.gov/Medicare/Demonstration-Projects/DemoProjectsEvalRpts/Downloads/PhysicianGroupPracticeFinalReport.pdf.

19. John K. Iglehart, "Assessing an ACO Prototype—Medicare's Physician Group Practice Demonstration," *New England Journal of Medicine* 364 (2011): 198–200.

20. CMS fact sheet, Medicare Physician Group Practice Demonstration ....

21. CMS fact sheet; RTI International, Marshfield Clinic Physician Group Practice Demonstration: Final Site Report, July 2006.

22. Douglas McCarthy, "Case Study: Improving Quality and Efficiency in Response to Pay-for-Performance Incentives Under the Medicare Physician Group Practice Demonstration," The Commonwealth Fund, March 12, 2007, accessed at http://www.commonwealthfund.org/Content/Innovations/Case-Studies/2007/Mar/Case-Study—Improving-Quality-and-Efficiency-in-Response-to-Pay-for-Performance-Incentives-Under-the.aspx.

23. RTI International, Geisinger Clinic Physician Group Practice Demonstration: Final Site Report, July 2006.

24. CMS Report to Congress on the Physician Group Practice Demonstration, 2009, 85–86.

25. Michael Trisolini, Jyoti Aggarwal, Musetta Leung, Gregory Pope, and John Kautter, "The Medicare Physician Group Practice Demonstration: Lessons Learned on Improving Quality and Efficiency in Health Care," *Commonwealth Fund*, February 2008, 20–35.

26. NCQA fact sheet, "Patient-Centered Medical Homes," accessed at http://www.ncqa.org/Portals/0/Public%20Policy/2013%20PDFS/pcmh%202011%20fact%20sheet.pdf.

27. CMS fact sheet, "Multi-Payer Advanced Primary Care Practice," accessed at http://innovation.cms.gov/initiatives/Multi-Payer-Advanced-Primary-Care-Practice/.

28. Blue Cross Shield Association fact sheet, "Patient-Centered Medical Home," http://www.bcbs.com/why-bcbs/patient-centered-medical-home/PCMH_FactSheet.pdf.

29. Daniel Fields, Elizabeth Leshen, and Kevita Patel, "Driving Quality Gains and Cost Savings Through Adoption of Medical Homes," *Health Affairs* 29, no. 5 (2010): 819–826.

30. Patient-Centered Primary Care Collaborative, "The Patient-Centered Medical Home: An Annual Update of the Evidence, 2012-2013," January 2014, accessed at http://www.pcpcc.org/sites/default/files/resources/4%20-%20Executive%20Summary%20and%20Evidence.pdf.

31. Patient-Centered Primary Care Collaborative, "Core Value, Community Connections: Care Coordination in the Medical Home," accessed at http://www.pcpcc.org/sites/default/files/media/carecoordination_pcpcc.pdf.

32. R. Antonelli, et al, "Providing a Medical Home: The Cost of Care Coordination Services in a Community-Based, General Pediatric Practice," *Pediatrics* 113, no. 5 (2004): 1522–1528.

33. Richard J. Baron and Emily Desnouee, "The Struggle to Support Patients' Effort to Change Their Unhealthy Behavior," *Health Affairs* 29 (May 2010): 953–955.

34. Mark A. Hall, Wenke Hwang, and Alison Snow Jones, "Model Safety-Net Programs Could Care For the Uninsured at One-Half the Cost of

Medicaid or Private Insurance," Health Affairs September 2011 vol. 30, no. 9, 1698-1707.

35. Bruce E. Landon, James M. Gill, Richard C. Antonelli, and Eugene C. Rich, "Prospects for Rebuilding Primary Care Using the Patient-Centered Medical Home," *Health Affairs* 29, no. 5 (2010): 827–834.

36. Robb Malone, "The Patient Centered Medical Home: Lessons learned from an academic medical center," UNC presentation, April 7, 2010, accessed at http://www.med.unc.edu/im/staff/documents/PCMH_April_2010

37. Mitesh S. Patel, Martin J. Arron, Thomas A. Sinsky, Eric H. Green, David W. Baker, Judith L. Bowen, and Susan Day, "Estimating the Staffing Infrastructure for a Patient-Centered Medical Home," *American Journal of Managed Care* 1, no.19 (June 21, 2013): N6, accessed at http://www.ajmc.com/publications/issue/2013/2013-1-vol19-n6/estimating-the-staffing-infrastructure-for-a-patient-centered-medical-home/1.

38. Ashok Rai, Paul Prichard, Richard Hodach, and Ted Courtemanche, "Using Physician-Led Automated Communications to Improve Patient Health," *Population Health Management* 14 (2011): accessed at http://info.phytel.com/rs/phytel/images/JournalPopulationHealth_UsingPhysician-LedAutomatedCommunications.pdf.

39. NCQA, "Standards and Guidelines for NCQA's Patient-Centered Medical Home (PCMH) 2014."

40. The Commonwealth Fund, Dartmouth Institute for Clinical Policy and Practice, and Patient Centered Primary Care Collaborative, "Better to Best" ... 20.

41. Ibid., 28.

42. Malone, "The Patient-Centered Medical Home."

43. Casalino, Gillies, Shortell, Schmittdiel, Bodenheimer, Robinson, Rundall, Oswald, Schauffler, and Wang, "External Incentives, Information Technology, and Organized Processes" ...

44. Trisolini, Aggarwal, Leung, Pope, and Kautter, "The Medicare Physician Group Practice Demonstration" ...

45. Phytel case studies, accessed at http://resources.phytel.com/case-study.

46. Ibid.

47. PCPCC, "Managing Populations, Maximizing Technology: Population Health Management in the Medical Neighborhood," October 2013, accessed at http://www.pcpcc.org/resource/managing-populations-maximizing-technology5.

48. Donald M. Berwick, Thomas W. Nolan, and John Whittington, "The Triple Aim: Care, Health and Cost," *Health Affairs*, May/June 2008, 759–769.

49. The Commonwealth Fund, Dartmouth Institute for Clinical Policy and Practice, and Patient Centered Primary Care Collaborative, "Better to Best" ... 20–26.

50. CMS, "CY 2015 Revisions to Payment Policies Under the Physician Fee Schedule," proposed rule, July 11, 2014, accessed at https://www.federalregister.gov/articles/2014/07/11/2014-15948/medicare-program-revisions-to-payment-policies-under-the-physician-fee-schedule-clinical-laboratory

51. Robert Pear, "Medicare to Start Paying Doctors Who Coordinate Needs of Chronically Ill Patients," New York Times, Aug. 16, 2014, accessed at http://www.nytimes.com/2014/08/17/us/medicare-to-start-paying-doctors-who-coordinate-needs-of-chronically-ill-patients.html?_r=0

Chapter 9

1. Debora Goetz Goldberg, Tishra Beeson, Anton J. Kuzel, Linda E. Love, and Mary C. Carver, "Team-Based Care: A Critical Element of Primary Care Practice Transformation," *Population Health Management* 16 (2013): 150–156.

2. Richard J. Baron and Emily Desnouee, "The Struggle to Support Patients' Effort to Change Their Unhealthy Behavior," *Health Affairs* 29 (May 2010): 953–955.

3. Thomas Bodenheimer, Amireh Ghorob, Rachel Willard-Grace, and Kevin Grumbach, "The 10 Building Blocks of High-Performing Primary Care," *Ann Fam Med* 12, no. 2 (March/April 2014): 166–171.

4. AAFP press release, "Six National Family Medicine Organizations Release 'Joint Principles: Integrating Behavioral Health Care Into

the Patient-Centered Medical Home," March 11, 2014, accessed at http://www.aafp.org/media-center/releases-statements/all/2014/joint-principles-pcmh.html.

5. Mitesh S. Patel, Martin J. Aaron, Thomas A. Sinsky, Eric H. Green, David W. Baker, Judith L. Bowen, and Susan Day, "Estimating the Staffing Infrastructure for a Patient-Centered Medical Home," *Am J Manag Care* 19, no. 6 (2013): 509–516.

6. Anthem Blue Cross and Blue Shield of Colorado, press release, "More than One-Third of Colorado's Primary Care Providers Working Under New Payment and Care Coordination Arrangement with Anthem," March 12, 2014, accessed at http://www.businesswire.com/news/home/20140312006098/en/One-Third-Colorado's-Primary-Care-Providers-Working-Payment#.Uz8d5BbiQwi.

7. Ken Terry, "Physician Payment Reform: What It Could Mean to Doctors—Part 1: Accountable Care Organizations," *Medscape*, Aug. 10, 2010, accessed at http://www.medscape.com/viewarticle/726537.

8. Institute for Health Technology Transformation, "Lean Health IT: The Next Step for Clinical and Business Intelligence," accessed at http://ihealthtran.com/iHT2LeanHealthIT.pdf?submissionGuid=082415b0-a22c-41fa-a683-c3fa0c0ee170.

9. Terry Young, Sally Brailsford, Con Connell, Ruth Davies, Paul Harper, and Jonathan H. Klein, "Using Industrial Processes to Improve Patient Care," *BMJ* 328 (2004): 162–4. Accessed at http://www.ncbi.nlm.nih.gov/pmc/articles/PMC314521/pdf/bmj32800162.pdf.

10. Steven J. Spear, "Fixing Healthcare from the Inside, Today," *Harvard Business Review*, September 2005.

11. Paul A. Nutting, Benjamin F. Crabtree, William L. Miller, Kurt C. Stange, Elizabeth Stewart, and Carlos Jaén, "Transforming Physician Practices to Patient-Centered Medical Homes: Lessons From the National Demonstration Project," *Health Affairs* 30 (March 2011): 446.

12. Ibid.

13. Institute for Health Technology Transformation, "Lean Health IT" …

14. Ibid.

15. Ken Terry, "Re-Engineer Your Practice—Starting Today," *Medical Economics*, Jan. 24, 2000, accessed at http://medicaleconomics.

modernmedicine.com/medical-economics/news/re-engineer-your-practice%C2%97starting-today.

16. Institute for Health Technology Transformation, "Lean Health IT" …

17. Ibid.

18. Maryjoan D. Ladden, Thomas Bodenheimer, Nancy W. Fishman, Margaret Flinter, Clarissa Hsu, Michael Parchman, and Edward H. Wagner, "The Emerging Primary Care Workforce: Preliminary Observations from the Primary Care Team: Learning From Effective Ambulatory Practices Project," *Academic Medicine* 88, no. 12 (Dec. 2013): 1830–1834.

19. Christine A. Sinsky, Rachel Willard-Grace, Andrew M. Schutzbank, Thomas A. Sinsky, David Margolius, and Thomas Bodenheimer, "In Search of Joy in Practice: A Report of 23 High-Functioning Primary Care Practices," *Annals of Family Medicine* 1 (2013): 272–278.

20. Goldberg, Beeson, Kuzel, Love, and Carver, "Team-Based Care" …

21. Patient-Centered Primary Care Collaborative, "Managing Populations, Maximizing Technology: Population Health Management in the Medical Neighborhood," October 2013, accessed at http://www.pcpcc.org/resource/managing-populations-maximizing-technology.

22. Sinsky, Willard-Grace, Schutzbank, Sinsky, Margolius, and Thomas Bodenheimer, "In Search of Joy in Practice"

23. Ibid.

24. Institute for Health Technology Transformation, "Lean Health IT" …

25. Ibid.

26. HIMSS press release, "HIMSS Introduces Health IT Value Suite to Realize the Value of Health IT," July 16, 2013, accessed at http://www.himss.org/News/NewsDetail.aspx?ItemNumber=21536.

27. Ashok Rai, Paul Prichard, Richard Hodach, and Ted Courtemanche, "Using Physician-Led Automated Communications to Improve Patient Health," *Population Health Management* 14, no. 4 (August 2011): 175–180.

Chapter 10

1. Anand K. Parekh, "Winning Their Trust," *New England Journal of Medicine* 364 (June 16, 2011): e51.

2. Thomas Pearson, "The Prevention of Cardiovascular Disease: Have We Really Made Progress?" *Health Affairs* 26, no. 1 (2007): 49–60.

3. Niteesh K. Choudhry, MD, PhD; Jerry Avorn, MD; Robert J. Glynn, ScD, PhD; Elliott M. Antman, MD; Sebastian Schneeweiss, MD, ScD; Michele Toscano, MS; Lonny Reisman, MD; Joaquim Fernandes, MS; Claire Spettell, PhD; Joy L. Lee, MS; Raisa Levin, MS; Troyen Brennan, MD, JD, MPH; and William H. Shrank, MD, "Full Coverage for Preventive Medications after Myocardial Infarction," *New England Journal of Medicine* (Nov. 14, 2011), doi:10.1056/NEJMsa1107913.

4. Lee Goldman, MD, and Arnold M. Epstein, MD, "Improving Adherence—Money Isn't the Only Thing," *New England Journal of Medicine* (Nov. 14, 2011), doi:10.1056/NEJMe1111558.

5. Pearson, "The Prevention of Cardiovascular Disease" …

6. David M. Lawrence, "How to Forge a High-Tech Marriage Between Primary Care and Population Health," *Health Affairs*, May 2010: 1004–1009.

7. Parekh, "Winning Their Trust" …

8. Annette M. O'Connor, John E. Wennberg, France Legare, Hilary A. Llewellyn-Thomas, Benjamin W. Moulton, Karen R. Sepucha, Andrea G. Sodano, and Jaime S. King, "Toward the 'Tipping Point': Decision Aids and Informed Patient Choice," *Health Affairs* 26, no. 3 (2007): 716–725.

9. Dorcas Mansell, MD, MPH; Roy M. Poses, MD; Lewis Kazis, ScD; and Corey A. Duefield, MPH, "Clinical Factors that Influence Patients' Desire for Participation in Decisions About Illness," *Archives of Internal Medicine* 160 (2000): 2991–2996.

10. American Academy of Family Physicians, American Academy of Pediatrics, American College of Physicians, and American Osteopathic Association, "Joint Principles of the Patient-Centered Medical Home," accessed at http://www.pcpcc.net/content/joint-principles-patient-centered-medical-home.

11. J. H. Hibbard, "Moving Toward a More Patient-Centered Health Care Delivery System," *Health Affairs*, October 2004, doi: 10.1377/hlthaff. var.133.

12. Ibid.

13. Center for Advancing Health, "A New Definition of Patient Engagement: What Is Patient Engagement and Why Is It Important?" (2010). Accessed at http://www.cfah.org/pdfs/CFAH_Engagement_Behavior_Framework_2010.pdf.

14. Judith H. Hibbard, Eldon R. Mahoney, Ronald Stock, and Martin Tusler. "Do Increases in Patient Activation Result in Improved Self-Management Behaviors?" *Health Services Research* 42, no. 4 (August 2007): 1443–1463.

15. Ibid.

16. J. O. Prochaska, John Norcross, and Carlo DiClemente, *Changing for Good* (New York: HarperCollins, 1995, 2002).

17. Karen Glanz, Barbara K. Rimer, and KJ. Viswanath, *Health Behavior and Health Education, 3rd Edition* (San Francisco: Jossey-Bass Inc., 2002).

18. Ibid.

19. Hibbard JH, Green J., Tusler M., "Improving the Outcomes of Disease Management by Tailoring Care to the Patient's Level of Activation," The American Journal of Managed Care. 2009 Jun;15(6):353-60.

20. B.J. Fogg, "A Behavior Model for Persuasive Design," paper presented at Persuasive '09 Conference, April 26-29, 2009, Claremont, Calif. Accessed at http://blog.hcilab.org/uui/files/2013/04/a40-fogg.pdf.

21. Peter J. Cunningham, Judith Hibbard, and Claire B. Gibbons, "Raising Low 'Patient Activation' Rates Among Hispanic Immigrants May Equal Expanded Coverage in Reducing Access Disparities," *Health Affairs* 30, no.10 (2011): 1888–1894.

22. Institute of Medicine, *Health Literacy: A Prescription to End Confusion* (Washington, DC: National Academy Press, 2004).

23. Ian Duncan, *Healthcare Risk Adjustment and Predictive Modeling* (Winstead, CT: ACTEX Publications, 2011).

24. Ashok Rai, Paul Prichard, Richard Hodach, and Ted Courtemanche, "Using Physician-Led Automated Communications to Improve Patient Health," *Journal of Population Health Management, vol. 14, 2011,* doi:10.1089/pop.2010.0033.

25. Peter Boland, Phil Polakoff, and Ted Schwab, "Accountable Care Organizations Hold Promise, But Will They Achieve Cost and

Quality Targets?" *Managed Care*, October 2010, accessed at http://www.managedcaremag.com/archives/1010/1010.ACOs.html.

26. Steven M. Schwartz, Brian Day, Kevin Wildenhaus, Anna Silberman, Chun Wang, and Jordan Silberman, "The Impact of an Online Disease Management Program on Medical Costs Among Health Plan Members," *American Journal of Health Promotion* 25, no. 2 (2010): 126–133.

27. Hibbard, "Moving Toward a More Patient-Centered System" …

28. Susannah Fox and Maeve Duggan, "Health Online 2013," Pew Research Center, Jan. 15, 2013, accessed at http://www.pewinternet.org/files/old-media//Files/Reports/PIP_HealthOnline.pdf.

29. Manhattan Research, "Cybercitizen Health v7.0" press release, Nov. 1, 2007.

30. Fox, "Peer-to-Peer Health Care," Pew Internet and American Life Project, Feb. 28, 2011, accessed at http://pewresearch.org/pubs/1908/online-health-information-peer-to-peer-patients-caregivers-chronic-conditions.

31. Emmi Solutions website, http://www.emmisolutions.com/patient_education_solutions.html.

32. S. Greenfield, S. H. Kaplan, J. E. Ware Jr., E. M. Yano, and H. J. Frank, "Patients' Participation in Medical Care: Effects on Blood Sugar Control and Quality of Life in Diabetics," *Journal of General Internal Medicine.* 3 (1988): 448–457.

33. C. M. Renders, G. D. Valk, S. J. Griffin, E. H. Wagner, J. T. Eijk Van, and W. J. Assendelft, "Interventions to Improve the Management of Diabetes in Primary Care, Outpatient, and Community Settings: A Systematic Review," *Diabetes Care* 24 (2001): 1821–1833.

34. Thomas Reinke, "Want to Change Patients' Behavior? Look to the Internet," *Managed Care*, July 2009, accessed at http://www.managedcaremag.com/archives/0907/0907.engagement.html.

35. HealthMedia website, http://www.healthmedia.com/.

36. Ken Terry, "Monitor Patients Online?" *Medical Economics*, July 23, 2001, accessed at http://www.modernmedicine.com/modernmedicine/article/articleDetail.jsp?id=118617.

37. E. A. Balas, S. Krishna, R. A. Kretschmer, T. R. Cheek, D. F. Lobach, and S. A. Boren, "Computerized Knowledge Management in Diabetes Care," *Medical Care* 42 (2004): 610–621.

38. M. C. Gibbons, R. F. Wilson, L. Samal, C. U. Lehmann, K. Dickersin, H. P. Lehmann, H. Aboumatar, J. Finkelstein, E. Shelton, R. Sharma, and E. B. Bass, *Impact of Consumer Health Informatics Applications*, Evidence Report/Technology Assessment No. 188. (Prepared by Johns Hopkins University Evidence-Based Practice Center under contract No. HHSA 290-2007-10061-I.) AHRQ Publication No. 09(10)-E019. Rockville, MD: Agency for Healthcare Research and Quality, October 2009.

39. Ken Terry, "VA Telehealth Lauded as Model Healthcare Program," *InformationWeek Healthcare*, Jan. 24, 2012, accessed at http://www. informationweek.com/mobile/va-telehealth-lauded-as-model-healthcare-program/d/d-id/1102433.

40. Jared Rhoads and Clive Flashman, "Teleservices for Better Health: Expanding the Horizon of Patient Engagement," CSC Global Institute for Emerging Healthcare Practices, accessed at http://assets1.csc.com/ health_services/downloads/CSC_TeleServices_for_Better_Health_ Expanding_the_Horizon_of_Patient_Engagement.pdf.

41. Pew Research Internet Project, "Mobile Technology Fact Sheet," accessed May 6, 2014, at http://www.pewinternet.org/fact-sheets/ mobile-technology-fact-sheet/.

42. Terry, "Mobile Apps: Proposed FDA Rule Will Disrupt Industry," *InformationWeek*, July 21, 2011, accessed at http://www. informationweek.com/news/healthcare/policy/231002336.

43. Terry, "Apple FaceTime May Be HIPAA Secure," *InformationWeek*, Oct. 21, 2011, accessed at http://www.informationweek.com/news/ healthcare/mobile-wireless/231900634.

44. Charlene C. Quinn, Michelle D. Shardell, Michael L. Terrin, Erik A. Barr, Shoshana H. Ballew, and Ann L. Gruber-Baldini, "Cluster-Randomized Trial of a Mobile Phone Personalized Behavioral Intervention for Blood Glucose Control," *Diabetes Care* 34, no. 9 (Sept. 2011): 1934–1942.

45. Jae-Hyoung Cho, Hye-Chung Lee, Dong-Jun Lim, Hyuk-Sang Kwon, and Kun-Ho Yoon, "Mobile Communication Using a Mobile

Phone with a Glucometer for Glucose Control in Type 2 Patients with Diabetes: As Effective as an Internet-based Glucose Monitoring System," *J Telemed Telecare* 15, no. 2 (March 2009): 77–82.

46. Anna-Lisa Silvestre, Valerie M. Sue, and Jill Y. Allen, "If You Build It, Will They Come? The Kaiser Permanente Model of Online Care," *Health Affairs* 28, no. 2 (2009): 334–344, doi:10.1377/hlthaff.28.2.334.

47. Paul C. Tang and David Lansky, "The Missing Link: Bridging the Provider-Patient Information Gap," *Health Affairs*, 24, no.5 (2005): 1290–1295, doi:10.1377/hlthaff.24.5.1290.

48. David W. Bates and Asaf Bitton, "The Future of Health Information Technology in the Patient-Centered Medical Home," *Health Affairs* 29, no. 4 (2010): 614–621, doi:10.1377/hlthaff.2010.0007.

49. Don Detmer, Meryl Bloomrosen, Brian Raymond, and Paul Tang, "Integrated Personal Health Records: Transformative Tools for Consumer-Centric Care," *BMC Medical Informatics and Decision Making* 8 (2008): 45, doi:10.1186/1472-6947-8-45.

50. Brian S. McGowan, Molly Wasko, Bryan Steven Vartabedian, Robert S. Miller, Desirae D Freiherr, and Maziar Abdolrasulnia, "Understanding the Factors That Influence the Adoption and Meaningful Use of Social Media by Physicians to Share Medical Information," *Journal of Medical Internet Research*, 14, no. 5 (2012): e117.

51. Pamela Lewis Dolan, "Nearly All Doctors Are Now on Social Media," *American Medical News*, Sept. 26, 2011, accessed at http://www.ama-assn.org/amednews/2011/09/26/bil20926.htm.

52. Terry, "Doctors, Patients Not Using The Same Social Spaces," *InformationWeek*, Sept. 30, 2011, accessed at http://www.informationweek.com/news/healthcare/patient/231602459.

Chapter 11

1. Stephen F. Jencks, Mark V. Williams, and Eric A. Coleman, "Rehospitalizations Among Patients in the Medicare Fee-for-Service Program," *New England Journal of Medicine* 360 (2009): 1418–1428.

2. Mark Taylor, "The Billion-Dollar U-Turn," *Hospitals & Health Networks*, May 2008.

3. Jencks, "Rehospitalization: The Challenge and the Opportunity," presentation, Integrated Healthcare Association conference, Oct. 2009.

4. Suni Kripalani, Amy T. Jackson, Jeffrey L. Schnipper, and Eric A. Coleman, "Promoting Effective Transitions of Care at Hospital Discharge," *Journal of Hospital Medicine* 2 (2007): 314–323.

5. Jencks, Williams, and Coleman, "Rehospitalizations Among Patients" ...

6. Neil Gold, "3 Readmissions to Reduce Now," *HealthLeaders Media*, March 15, 2011, accessed at http://www.healthleadersmedia.com/content/COM-263665/3-Readmissions-to-Reduce-Now.html.

7. CMS, "Readmissions Reduction Program," accessed at http://www.cms.gov/Medicare/Medicare-Fee-for-Service-Payment/AcuteInpatientPPS/Readmissions-Reduction-Program.html.

8. Julia James, "Health Policy Brief: Medicare Hospital Readmissions Reduction Program," *Health Affairs*, Nov. 12, 2013, accessed at http://healthaffairs.org/healthpolicybriefs/brief_pdfs/healthpolicybrief_102.pdf.

9. Ken Terry, "Patient Safety Front and Center," *Hospitals & Health Networks*, July 2011.

10. CMS, "Bundled Payments for Care Improvement Initiative Fact Sheet," Jan. 30, 2014, accessed at http://www.cms.gov/Newsroom/MediaReleaseDatabase/Fact-Sheets/2014-Fact-sheets-items/2014-01-30-2.html.

11. Rich Daly and Jessica Zigmond, "CMS Issues Proposed ACO Regulation," *Modern Healthcare*, March 31, 2011.

12. Kripalani, Jackson, Schnipper, and Coleman, "Promoting Effective Transitions of Care" ...

13. Ibid.

14. Susan Baird Kanaan, "Homeward Bound: Nine Patient-Centered Programs Cut Readmissions," California Healthcare Foundation report, September 2009.

15. Edwin D. Boudreaux, Sunday Clark, and Carlos A. Camargo, "Telephone Follow-Up after the Emergency Department Visit: Experience with Acute Asthma," *Annals Emergency Medicine* 35 (June 2000): 555–563.

16. Gail Neilsen and Peg Bradke, presentation at Institute for Healthcare Improvement conference, July 13, 2011.

17. Kripalani, Jackson, Schnipper, and Coleman, "Promoting Effective Transitions of Care" …

18. Ibid.

19. Kripalani S., LeFevre F., Phillips CO, Williams MV, Basaviah P, Baker DW, "Deficits in Communication and Information Transfer Between Hospital-Based and Primary Care Physicians: Implications for Patient Safety and Continuity of care," *JAMA* 297, no. 8 (2007): 831–841.

20. Roy CL, Poon EG, Karson AS, Ladak-Merchant Z, Johnson RE, Maviglia SM, Gandhi TK, "Patient Safety Concerns Arising from Test Results That Return after Hospital Discharge," *Annals Internal Medicine* 143, no. 2 (2005): 121–128.

21. Kripalani, Jackson, Schnipper, and Coleman, "Promoting Effective Transitions of Care" …

22. Ibid.

23. Society of Hospital Medicine website, Project BOOST, accessed at http://www.hospitalmedicine.org/AM/Template.cfm?Section= Home&TEMPLATE=/CM/HTMLDisplay.cfm&CONTENTID= 27659.

24. Physician Consortium for Performance Improvement, "Care Transitions Performance Measurement Set," June 2009.

25. Transitions of Care Consensus Policy Statement American College of Physicians-Society of General Internal Medicine-Society of Hospital Medicine-American Geriatrics Society-American College of Emergency Physicians-Society of Academic Emergency Medicine, *Journal of General Internal Medicine* 24, no. 8 (Aug. 2009): 971–6.

26. Phytel presentation, "IHI and PCMH Perspectives."

27. Peg Bradke and Gail Nielsen, "Getting Started," presentation at Institute of Healthcare Improvement seminar, "Reducing Avoidable Readmissions by Improving Transitions of Care," July 13, 2011.

28. Kanaan, "Homeward Bound," op. cit.

29. Eric A. Coleman, Carla Parry, Sandra Chalmers, and Sung-Joon Min, "The Care Transitions Intervention: Results of a Randomized Controlled Trial," *Archives of Internal Medicine* 166, no. 17 (2006): 1822–8.

30. Ibid.

31. Eric A. Coleman, Jodi D. Smith, Janet C. Frank, Sung-Joon Min, Carla Parry, and Andrew M. Kramer, "Preparing Patients and Caregivers to

Participate in Care Delivered Across Settings: The Care Transitions Intervention," *Journal of the American Geriatric Society* 52 (2004): 1817–1825.

32. Kanaan, "Homeward Bound."

33. Ibid.

34. Naylor MD, Brooten DA, Campbell RL, et al., "Advanced practice nurse directed transitional care reduced readmission or death in elderly patients admitted to hospital with heart failure," Journal of the American Geriatric Society 2004;52:675–84.

35. Vicky Dudas, Thomas Bookwalter, Kathleen M. Keer, and Stephen Z. Pantilat, "The Impact of Follow-Up Telephone Calls to Patients after Hospitalization," *American Journal of Medicine*, 111, no. 9, supplement 2: 26–30.

36. *Journal of Emergency Medicine*, 6 (1988).

37. Nielsen and Bradke presentation, op. cit.

38. Kripalani, Jackson, Schnipper, and Coleman, "Promoting Effective Transitions of Care" …

39. Emmi website, www.emmisolutions.com.

40. Mari Edlin, "Digital Health Coaching Brings Care Management to Everyday Life," *Managed Healthcare Executive*, Jan 1, 2011.

41. Physician Consortium for Performance Improvement, "Care Transitions Performance Measurement Set" …

42. Kripalani, Jackson, Schnipper, and Coleman, "Promoting Effective Transitions of Care" …

43. Physician Consortium for Performance Improvement, "Care Transitions Performance Measurement Set" …

44. Kathleen Louden, "Creating a Better Discharge Summary: Is Standardization the Answer?" *ACP Hospitalist*, March 2009.

45. Janice Simmons, "Direct Project Gets Widespread Industry Support," Fierce EMR, March 24, 2011, accessed at http://www.fierceemr.com/story/direct-project-gets-widespread-industry-support/2011-03-24.

About the Author

Richard Hodach, MD, is the author of Provider-Led Population Health Management. Dr. Hodach, Phytel's chief medical officer and vice president of Clinical Product Strategy, has long been recognized as a leader of population health management strategies. He is responsible for providing strategic direction and clinical expertise for the development of Phytel's solutions. Dr. Hodach is a regular contributor to prestigious peer-review journals such as AJMC, Journal of Population Health Management, published by the Healthcare Financial Management Association, Group Practice Journal, and more. He was instrumental in the CMS Innovation Award of a $20.75 million grant which Phytel, VHA Inc. and TransforMED received from The Center for Medicare & Medicaid Innovation (CMMI). In addition to his leadership position at Phytel, Dr. Hodach also serves on the board of directors of the American Board of Medical Quality, and will also serve as chair. Before joining Phytel, he held senior leadership positions at Matria Healthcare and Accordant, and cofounded MED.I.A. Dr. Hodach has a PhD in Pathology and an MD with board certification in neurology and electrodiagnosis, as well as a master's degree in public health.

Acknowledgements

I would like to thank the extraordinary group of people below who made significant contributions to this book. Without them, this book would certainly not exist.

Bill Buck
Ted Courtemanche
Patrick Flynn
Jerry Green
Karen Handmaker
Jon Mark Harmon
Jeffrey Havlock
Guy Mansueto
Adam McCoy
Jorge Miranda
Russell Olsen
Marina Pascali
Kristy Sanders
Steve Schelhammer
Carly Sheppard-Knoll
Ken Terry

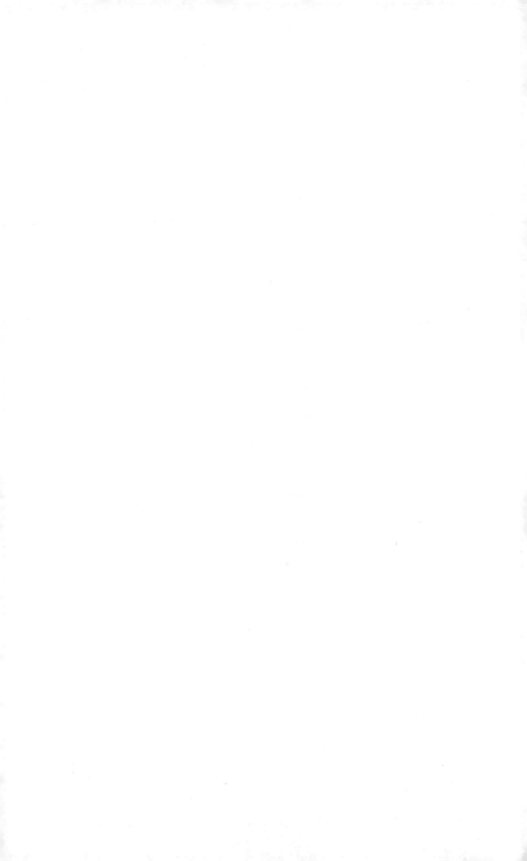

CPSIA information can be obtained
at www.ICGtesting.com
Printed in the USA
FSOW02n1746031115
12916FS

9 781496 941749